Dr. Mikao Usui and Frank Arjava Petter

The Original
Reiki Handbook
of Dr. Mikao Usui

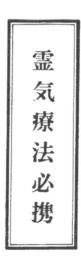

霊
気
療
法
必
携

For the first time available outside of Japan:

The Traditional Usui Reiki Ryoho
Treatment Positions and Numerous Reiki Techniques
for Health and Well-Being

Foreword by William Lee Rand

Translated by Christine M. Grimm

LOTUS PRESS
SHANGRI-LA

Important Note:
The information presented in this book has been carefully researched and passed on according to our best knowledge and conscience. However, the author and publisher assume no liability whatsoever for damages of any kind that occur directly from the application or use of the statements in this book. This information is meant as further education for interested parties. The methods of healing and exercises listed in this book are no substitute for consulting a physician or naturopath. They are meant to support the healing process as an additional treatment. The laws of the USA permit the practice of medicine only by registered physicians and healing practitioners who have been trained in accordance with the law.

Frank Arjava Petter

In 1993 he brought Reiki back to the land of its origin and was the first Westener to teach the Reiki Master/Teacher Degree in Japan. Together with his Japanese wife Chetna, he traced back the various Reiki streams to their roots, the original system of Dr. Mikao Usui and discovered along with exciting historical facts, new and fascinating healing techniques from the origins of this fantastic system.

Frank Arjava Petter currently teaches together with his wife Chetna original Reki techniques in seminars and lectures. His books *Reiki Fire* and *Reiki—The Legacy of Dr. Usui* have already become international bestsellers.

Fifth English Edition 2011
© by Lotus Press
Box 325, Twin Lakes, WI 53181, USA
The Shangri-La Series is published in cooperation
with Schneelöwe Verlagsberatung, Federal Republic of Germany
©1998 by Windpferd Verlagsgesellschaft mbH, Aitrang, Germany
All rights reserved
Translated by Christine M. Grimm
Cover design by Kuhn Graphik, Digitales Design, Zurich, by using a picture of P.T Grigg
Interior illustrations: Shouya P.T. Grigg,
Picture of Dr. Usui on page 6: by T. Oishi
Drawings by: Peter Ehrhardt
Calligraphies: Shunyu Chikai (on page 9), Japanese typography: by Chetna Kobayashi
ISBN 978-0-9149-5557-3
Library of Congress Control Number 99-76564
Printed in USA

Expression of Thanks

During the past few years, a feeling of gratitude has grown in my heart, a deep thankfulness toward every moment of my life. A thankfulness toward all the people and the situations that I have encountered on my path. A thankfulness without a goal and without a source.

Yet, I would like to express my heartfelt thanks to a few friends, without whose assistance this work would have not been completed: first, my wife Chetna for her love and inexhaustible energy that she shares with me every day of our lives; and T. Oishi and Shizuko Akimoto for their boundless trust. The Windpferd team for its competent and loving support on the professional, as well as the personal, level. Walter Lübeck, who encourages me time and again to keep on researching; Christine M. Grimm for her lovely translation from German to English; Shunyu Chikai for the radiant calligraphy on the next page; Shouya P.T. Grigg for the wonderful photos that depict the spirit of Reiki so well. My loving thanks also to our supermodel Kumiko Kondo and to Masano Kobayashi, my mother-in-law, for the transcription of the Usui Memorial.

This book is also dedicated to the very special memory of Fumio Ogawa, who died in the summer of 1998: In the name of the world-wide Reiki community, I thank him posthumously for all the information that he so open-heartedly shared with us.

And naturally a sincere thank-you to all of you, my dear readers, for the thousands of letters, love, and suggestions with which you have showered me.

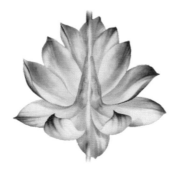

Foreword

A powerful process is taking place on the planet that is destined to bring about the peace we so desperately need. The end of the cold war, the improvement in global communications and the developing understanding that all the people of the world can and must work together if the planet is to survive is acting to transform our most basic concepts. A greater feeling of security along with the acceptance that the world has a viable future is encouraging people to create positive changes that support a peaceful planet.

Part of this process involves dispelling old restrictive beliefs and replacing them with the truth. As this happens people are gaining freedom and are in a better position to create a more desirable world.

We see this process taking place in the world of Reiki. The original western version of Reiki has been questioned and people are discovering more accurate information about its history and practice from which all can benefit. Over the past several years Arjava Petter and his Japanese wife Chetna Kobayashi have been uncovering important information concerning the origin and practice of Reiki in Japan. In spite of opposition from those in the west who would benefit by maintaining the status quo, they have proceeded with their research and with the publication of this book, are sharing their most important discoveries. The fact that Usui sensei had a training manual he gave to all his Reiki students is of paramount importance. It demonstrates that Reiki is not an oral tradition and that written material is an important part of the practice. Learning about the philosophy and practical exercises taught by Usui sensei creates an important level of understanding that connects us more strongly to the essence of Reiki. It gives us a better grasp of who Usui sensei was and helps improve the quality of healing we use for ourselves and others. Because of this, it is easy to understand why the translation and distribution of this manual is the most significant contribution to the practice of Usui Reiki since it was first brought to the west in 1938. This information will create a powerful shift in the Reiki community, helping to bring unity at the same time it improves the authenticity of the practice as well as the value it offers. I am sure that all who read this book will benefit in many ways.

William Lee Rand
September, 1999
The International Center for Reiki Training, Southfield, MI

Table of Contents

Dedication

Dedicated to Mikao Usui in love and gratitude

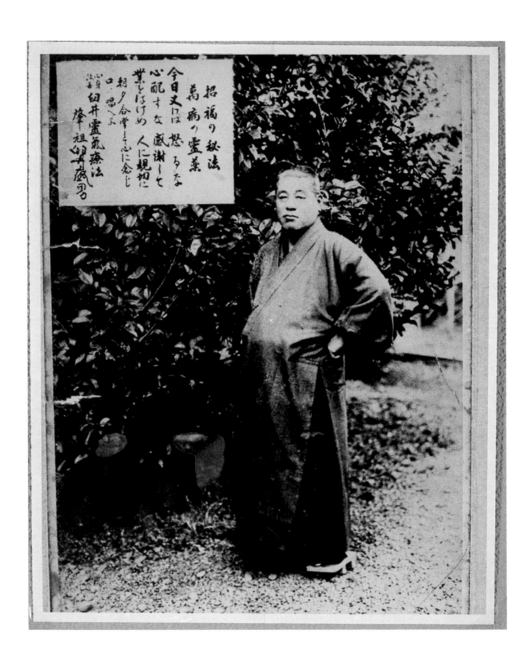

Introduction

Dear Reiki friends, this time I would like to once again introduce something "new" from Reiki's country of origin: the practical section of the *Usui Reiki Ryoho Hikkei*, in which Dr. Usui gives a detailed description of the hand positions for the treatment of certain body areas and health disorders. When my wife Chetna and I received the handbook, in addition to a few other historical Japanese Reiki writings from T. Oishi in the summer of 1997, we decided to only publish this section after a thorough investigation of it. We also wanted to wait until we had had enough personal experiences with this aspect of the Reiki work, which was new to us at that time.

Now we don't want to keep it from you any longer.

The hand positions described in Dr. Usui's handbook are considerably more extensive than those that we have learned to use and love in the West.

However, by publishing this book I do not mean to depict the twelve Western hand positions as "false." They remain the basis for a whole-body treatment. They are certainly helpful and important, especially for beginners on the Reiki path. This current book is meant to take us back to the roots of Reiki. Moreover, it is also meant to increase and intensify our understanding of the Reiki power.

Dr. Usui's handbook includes a wonderful diversity of information. In my opinion, this information can only be comprehended to the full extent of its power when it is also presented in a visual manner.

This is why Chetna and I decided to add photos of the hand positions, as well as drawings of the described body areas, in order to give you a handbook that is clearly understandable and easy to put into practice. You can also consult it for advice in your Reiki practice. I have added the first four chapters—"The Buddhist Background of Reiki," "The Three Pillars of Reiki," "The Breath," and "Dr. Usui's Techniques of Healing" in order to present the foundations of Dr. Usui's work in the most complete way possible. The information contained here comes from an interview with Dr. Usui that I published in my last book, as well as conversations between Shizuko Akimoto and Fumio Ogawa, and further Japanese Reiki sources.

Reiki was taught and learned very intensively under Dr. Usui. The students met once a week to meditate, apply Reiki together, and practice scanning the body until they succeeded in reaching a type of energetic diagnosis. If this was the case, the corresponding areas of the body were treated immediately. Some Reiki students were immediately successful in doing this, while others required a few weeks, months, or years. The Reiki power naturally finds its own paths, precisely where it is needed. However, this does not exclude the possibility of the people giving the treatment following their own inspiration with their hands. A Western Reiki treatment is a type of large-scale treatment; the Japanese, intuitive treatment is specifically directed: the more precise we work, the better the results will naturally be.

In Japan, the Reiki path is seen as a course of life that is followed through many decades to the end of a person's days. A student in Japan sometimes only attained the Second Reiki Degree after ten or twenty years of practice. And the majority of the students never achieved the higher levels. They were and always remained students.

Here in the West, Reiki has developed in a direction that more closely corresponds with our culture. People meet on one day or a weekend to learn the First Degree. There often isn't even enough time to learn to listen to their bodies, their hands, and their intuition. Although this is a shame, it simply isn't possible for many Western Reiki students and teachers to come into contact with this energy in any other way. Life in the fast lane of Western civilization—and here I include the modern Japanese way of life as well—takes place at high speeds. Many of us no longer have the time and want to have whatever we have cast our eyes on immediately, at this very moment.

I don't want to suggest turning back the clock. We have to face the demands of the present. And these twelve hand positions in particular are an important tool that can be learned quickly. With their help, each of us can practice on our own at home, without instructions and without the fear of doing something "wrong." These hand positions cover the entire system of the endocrine glands, as well as all of the inner organs. They energize the human being on a number of levels at the same time:

• On the physical level through the warmth of the hands
• On the mental level through the thoughts or Reiki symbols
• On the emotional level through the love that flows with them
• On the energetic level through the presence of the initiated person, as well as the Reiki power itself.

A further advantage of the twelve hand positions is that people who practice treating themselves every day learn how to use the Reiki energy. If you have ever received a whole-body treatment from loving hands or treated yourself for several weeks, this experience will remain with you long after it is over.

Intuitive Reiki by Dr. Usui is different: It asks that we free ourselves of the rules. Rules are meant to give us support. The moment that they begin to hinder us, they no longer fulfill their purpose.

The best approach is to gradually start integrating the techiques and information described in this book into your own practice of Reiki—and the clients will love your hands.

Many of you have certainly worked in an intuitive manner for a long time. I am happy for you—and with you—that we now have the "official" permission from Dr. Mikao Usui to do this!

From the depths of my heart, I wish all of you much enjoyment and pleasure in reading and exploring these new, wonderful possibilities in the practice. This is what they are meant for!

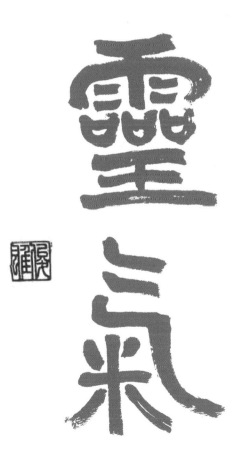

The old Reiki-Kanji, as it was written prior to 1940

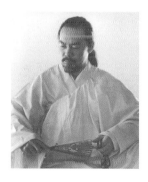

A calligraphy by Shunyu Chikai, born in 1950, who was ordinated as a Shingon monk in 1973. He founded the Shakya-yoga-ashram in Marugame, Shikoku, Japan, where he teaches meditations techniques and Reiki to his students.

The Buddhist Background of Reiki

The inscription on Dr. Usui's grave tells us that he experienced the Reiki power during a twenty-one day fasting retreat on Mount Kurama.

The monk Gantei, a student of Ganjin (the founder of the Toshodaiji Temple in Nara) established the imposing Kurama temple in the year 770, after undergoing a deep religious experience there. Until 1949, Kurama Temple was connected with Tendai Buddhism; then it became the headquarters of the Kurama-Kokyo Sect*. In the office of the temple, we were assured that twenty-one day fasting/meditation retreats had never been held there. However, it was insinuated that one individual or another might have carried these out on his own, especially in earlier times. Thanks to its size, its strong energy, and its giant ancient stand of cedars, Mount Kurama offers the perfect setting for meditation and the search for the self. Today, it is possible to spend a day and a night meditating and writing mantras at the Kurama Temple by registering there in advance of your visit.

Moreover, there are still a few small, beautiful Shinto shrines on and near Mount Kurama. The Kubune Jinja (shrine), which lies beneath the Kurama on the street to Kyoto, should be mentioned in particular. Shintoism and Buddhism are deeply intertwined with each other in Japan, so it isn't always easy for laypeople to determine whether they are in a Buddhist temple or a Shinto shrine. In any case, Kurama is worth the journey!

Dr. Usui was a Buddhist, so I would like to make a brief digression into Japanese history, as well as the concepts that strongly influenced Dr. Usui, on the following pages in a short summary. It would certainly be possible to write an entire book on this topic, but that would go beyond the meaning and purpose of this work, as well as exceeding my knowledge of Buddhism.

* The word "sect" means a "small community of faith" here.

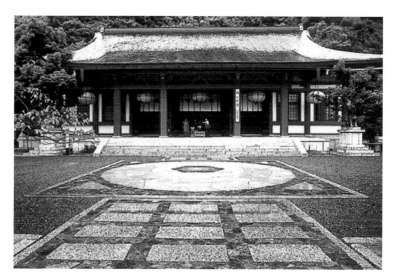

(The address of the Kurama Temple: Kurama Honmachi, Sakyo-Ku, Kyoto, Japan. Tel: 0081-75-7412003. The best way to reach the temple is by taking either the subway or the bus to the Demachiyanagi Station from the central train station in Kyoto. Then take a cozy train, the Eizan-Kurama line, to Kurama until the final station. From there, you can walk to the entrance gate of the Kurama Temple in five minutes.)

The Origin and the Goal

Esoteric Tantric Buddhism came to Japan in the early ninth century through the Japanese monk Kukai (Kobo Daishi, 774-835) and Saicho (Dengyo Daishi, 767-822), who had studied in China.

Kukai was a student of Huikuo (Japanese: Keika, 746-805), a student of the Indian monk Amoghavajra who was in turn a student of the famous Indian teacher Vajrabodhi. Both Indians lived in the Tahsingshan Temple in Ch'angan, the current center for the *Shensi Buddhist Association* in China. After the death of his teacher, Kukai returned to Japan and taught what he had learned in China. He became the founder of *Shingon* Buddhism.

Saicho studied on the Tien-tai Mountain in China. After his return, he became the founder of Tendai Buddhism, with its headquarters in Kyoto.

In Japan, both of these schools are often given the mutual name of Mikkyo.

The patron saint of esoteric Buddhism in Japan is Dainichi Nyorai (Mahavairocana Tathagata), and the most important and holiest writings are the *Dainichi-Kyo* ((*Mahavairocana Sutra*) and the *Kongocho Gyo* (*Vajrasekhara Sutra*). Here is Dainichi Nyorai's beautiful mantra:

Visualize:

The entire universe consists of six elements.
My body, which is made of six elements, is the body of the Dainichi Nyorai.
I am filled with whole, perfect, and unlimited life.
The five wisdoms are embodied in boundless, great compassion.
Nyorai's great compassion penetrates me.
I am included in Nyorai's great compassion.
I am blessed, I am blessed

(From Kaji-Empowerment and Healing in Esoteric Buddhism, by Ven. Ryuko Oda ISBN 4-905757-23-1 C0015)

In brief, the goal of esoteric Buddhism is *Shunyata*, emptiness. This emptiness is not a negative state of absence; instead, it should be understood as the transcendence of duality. At the moment in which the "self" is no longer distinct from "the other," the unity of the whole has once again been restored. The "self" only exists in our imagination, in our mind. We create the ego and the world with our thoughts. Our natural state of being is emptiness, unsullied by attributes, by the past and the future.

For many of us, this goal is also connected with Reiki in a similar way: experiencing oneness with the cosmos, returning back to the origin, to unity.

In my opinion, the most beautiful description of this state beyond duality is written in the so-called Heart Sutra (*Prajnaparamita Hridayam Sutra*)**.

** from *Buddhist Scriptures,*
by Edward Conze,
Penguin Classics,
ISBN 0-14-044088-7

The Heart Sutra

1 The Invocation.
Homage to the perfection of wisdom, the lovely, the holy!

2 The Foreword.
Avalokita, the holy Lord and Bodhisattva, was moving in the deep course of wisdom which has gone beyond. He looked down from on high, he beheld but five heaps, and he saw that in their own-being they were empty.

3. The Dialectic of Emptiness. First Stage.
Here, O Sariputra, form is emptiness, and the very emptiness is form; emptiness does not differ from form, and form does not differ from emptiness; whatever is form, that is emptiness, whatever is emptiness, that is form. The same is true of feelings, perceptions, impulses, and consciousness.

4 The Dialectic of Emptiness. Second Stage.
Here, O Sariputra, all dharmas are marked with emptiness; they are not produced or stopped, not defiled or immaculate, not deficient or complete.

5 The Dialectic of Emptiness. Third Stage.
Therefore, O Sariputra, in emptiness there is no form nor feeling, nor perception, nor impulse, nor consciousness; no eye, ear, nose, tongue, body, mind; no forms, sounds, smells, tastes, touchable, or objects of mind; no sight-organ-element, and so forth, until we come to: no-mind-consciousness-element; there is no ignorance, no extinction of ignorance, and so forth until we come to: there is no decay and death, no extinction of decay and death; there is no suffering, no origination, no stopping, no path; there is no cognition, no attainment, and no non attainment.

6 The Concrete Embodyment and Practical Basis of Emptiness.
Therefore, O Sariputra, it is because of his indifference to any kind of personal attainment that a Bodhisattva, through having relied on the perfection of wisdom, dwells without thought coverings. In the absence of thought-coverings, he has not been made to tremble, he has overcome what can upset, and in the end he attains Nirvana.

7 Full Emptiness Is the Basis also of Buddhahood
All those who appear as Buddhas in the three periods of time fully awake to the utmost, right and perfect enlightenment because they have relied on the perfection of wisdom.

8 The Teaching Brought within Reach of the Comparatively Unenlightened
Therefore one should know the Prajnaparamita as the great spell, the spell of great knowledge, the utmost spell, the unequalled spell, allayer of all suffering, in truth—for what could be wrong?
By the Prajnaparamita has this spell been delivered. It runs like this: Gone, Gone, Gone beyond, Gone alltogether beyond. O, what an awakening. All Hail! This completes the Heart of Perfect Wisdom.

---

* Here the so-called aggregates: form, emotion, perception, will or impulse and consciousness. WIth the help of these five aggregates our mind gives birth to the ego-consciousness

The vertical lines are read from right to left and from top to bottom:

1st column: Body and spirit will develop better with the Usui Reiki Ryoho teaching
2nd column: The secret law to invite happiness
3rd column: Spiritual medicine against all illness
4th – 9th column: The five Reiki principles

心身改善 臼井靈氣療法教義

招福の秘法

萬病の靈薬

今日丈けは怒るな

心配すな感謝して

業をはげめ人に親切に

朝夕合掌して

心に念じ

口に唱へよ

The Three Pillars of Reiki

Besides the five Reiki principles Dr. Usui taught his Reiki system, which is based on three pillars: *Gassho*, *Reiji-Ho*, and *Chiryo*.

Gassho

Gassho literally means "two hands coming together" and Dr. Usui taught a meditation by the name of Gassho Meditation. This meditation was practiced each time at the beginning of his Reiki workshops/meetings. It is meant to be practiced for 20-30 minutes after getting up and/or in the evening before going to sleep. Gassho can be done alone or in a group. Group meditations are a wonderful experience since the energy increases far beyond the sum of the individual participant's energies.

The Gassho Meditation is so simple that individuals of any age can do it. Whether we like it or not is another question. For my part, I love it very much and can also warmly recommend it. After three days of practice, you will know on the basis of your feelings whether it is "right" for you. Then, if possible, you should practice it every day for at least three months.

However, if after one or two days you have a feeling of restlessness, irritability, or some other form of annoyance, this meditation may possibly not be suitable for you. Not every medicine works for each patient. Then you can simply try it again after a few weeks.

Many people who are experienced in meditation know how difficult it is to forget everything and let go of our rational mind and the inner dialog. However, we tend to forget especially when we want to remember something! My tip is to disidentify yourself from your thoughts and feelings during meditation, as well as from your senses, but don't close yourself off to them. Whenever we try to close ourselves, this is when the inner dialog really starts up.

- When doing Gassho, sit down with closed eyes and hands placed together in front of your chest. Focus your entire attention at the point where the two middle fingers meet. Try to forget everything else. If you begin to think about lunch or the coming day during this meditation, observe the thought and then let it go.
- This is not a matter of achieving something. Relax as well as you can relax. Then return to the point where your middle fingers meet.

- If it is painful for you to hold your hands folded together in front of your chest for twenty minutes, let your hands (keeping them together) slowly sink down to your lap into a comfortable position and continue to meditate.
- Energy phenomena may also occur, such as your hands or backbone becoming very warm: Observe this but don't let yourself be influenced by it. Always return your focus to your two middle fingers.
- If you must change your sitting position, then move in slow motion: deliberately and consciously. In my experience, it is easier to meditate when the spinal column is as straight as possible, and the head doesn't tilt either forward, backward, or to the side. Imagine that your head is attached to a balloon filled with helium, which gently keeps it in the perfect position. If you have back problems or aren't used to sitting, I recommend that you sit on a chair with a back, with a few pillows behind you, or with your back leaned against the wall. There are basically no objections to meditating while lying down except that it invites us to fall asleep.

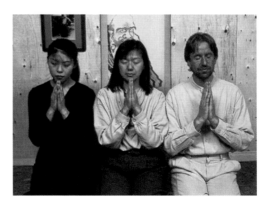

In Japan during Dr. Usui's time, people naturally sat on their knees, as we see in the photo. But since this seated position is uncomfortable for many of us, a meditation bench or chair will do.

Reiji-Ho

Translated into English, *Reiji* means "indication of the Reiki power." *Ho* means "methods." (In Hawayo Takata's journal, this method, as well as the breathing technique in the following chapter, was mentioned in an entry of May 1936.)

Reiji-Ho consists of three short rituals that are carried out before each treatment:

- Fold your hands in front of your chest in the Gassho posture and close your eyes. Now connect with the Reiki power. This is very simple: Ask the Reiki power to flow through you. Within a few seconds, you will notice how it flows. Perhaps you will feel it enter through your crown chakra or you may notice it first in your heart or in your hands. It doesn't matter in which part of your body the indication first occurs. If you have mastered Second Degree Reiki, you can use the distance-healing symbol to connect with the Reiki power. Repeat the wish three times in your mind that Reiki may flow, then send the mental-healing symbol and seal it all with the power symbol. Both symbols are learned during the Second Degree Reiki course. As soon as you feel the energy, continue on to the next step.
- Pray for the recovery and/or health of the patient on all levels. Here I would like to emphasize that we often do not even know what is "good" or "bad" for our patients. Put the terms "recovery" and "health" in the hands of the Reiki power and become a tool for it.
- Now hold your folded hands in front of your third eye and ask the Reiki power to guide your hands to where the energy is needed.

At first glance, this technique may seem strange to some of you, contradicting what you have learned about Reiki. However, on the basis of my own experience with this technique, I can't encourage all of you enough to experiment with it. I am not a very visually oriented person; consequently, it isn't easy for me to see on the etheric level. Because of this, for many years I used a pendulum to find the negatively charged areas of the body. But since I have started practicing Reiji, I no longer need the pendulum.

Your hands know what is happening, so learn to trust them. Intuition, some of you may think, is something that must be developed and learned. But the situation is actually quite different in reality: We are all basically intuitive. We just have to learn to listen to the inspiration that is already there and "translate" it correctly. How you get in touch with your intuition and in what area it manifests itself is different for each individual. I am a great fan of music, which makes me an auditory type of person. I perceive my surroundings intensively with the sense of hearing and "hear" my inspiration; for example, right now I'm hearing this text as I write it.

In case you are still uncertain, find out in which life situations your intuition has already functioned well. There is certain to be an area—perhaps (like my wife) while showering, cooking, taking a walk, or driving the car. Then carry this ability into other areas of your life as well.

But now back to the work with and on a client: Perhaps you see where an energy block is in the body or on the subtle plane. Perhaps you feel or smell it?

It is simple to carry out the Reiji ritual in a mechanical way, but that isn't the point of it. Try to get involved with your whole heart each time you do it, just like the very first time. The most important components involved in this are love and attention. These two qualities will show your client and you the path to healing and well-being.

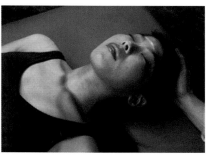

Chiryo (crown chakra)

Chiryo

Chiryo means "treatment" in English. In Dr. Usui's day, treatment was naturally given in a Japanese way. The patient lay on the floor, either on a futon (cotton mattress) or on a tatami mat (rush straw mattress).

• The practitioner kneeled next to the client. Fortunately, there is nothing to be said against giving a treatment on a massage table!

• The person giving the treatment holds his/her dominant hand above the client's crown chakra (see photo) and waits until there is an impulse or inspiration, which the hand then follows.

• During the treatment, the treatment-giver gives free rein to his/her hands, touches painful areas of the body until they no longer hurt or until the hands lift from the body on their own and find a new area to treat.

Dr. Usui used many different healing techniques, and some of them are described in more detail in the chapter on "Dr. Usui's Healing Techniques," which starts on page 25.

I understand the three pillars of Reiki in the following manner:
1. With the *Gassho Meditation*, we bring ourselves into a meditative state, a state of oneness with the universe. We clean the house before the

guest—in this case, Reiki energy—can come in. In India, Gassho is called *Namaste*, which means "I greet the divine within you." Once we have attained this state, we can take the next step. The Gassho Meditation is practiced daily so that it can be done before the treatment and during the Reiji, for which the hands are also folded in front of the chest. It helps the heart to be attuned with the treatment. It also teaches us to associate folding our hands in front of the chest with meditation. When we fold our hands and close our eyes, we automatically fall into a state of meditation.

2. *Reiji* can only be practiced effectively when the ego is temporarily switched off through meditation. At first glance, Reiji looks like a purposeful act; but in reality, we devote ourselves to the Reiki energy with Reiji. And devotion has no goal. The spiritual attitude in Reiji is: Thy will be done. After all, we are not the ones who accomplish the healing: Instead, it occurs at best through us.

A little pre-treatment ritual may help some of you. Wash your hands under cold, running water and briefly rinse out your mouth. In the treatment room, sit or stand comfortably in the Gassho posture. Close your eyes and let go of your worries, thoughts, and feelings. Now begin with Reiji.

3. Once you have begun the treatment, *Chiryo*, you no longer need to be concerned about healing or any other treatment goal.

Touching and Healing

If your hands are cold, rub them together vigorously a number of times to warm them up. When you place them on a part of the body, cold hands can temporarily take warmth away from it. Even when we treat a person with fever, we don't want to draw out the fever and saddle ourselves with it. There are possibilities of drawing illness out of the body and then giving them to plants, for example. However, these methods are not completely safe and should therefore only be carried out by those who know exactly what they are doing.

I sometimes hear that people have had energy taken away from them during a Reiki treatment. Something is wrong with this kind of treatment. In my experience, those who have been properly initiated into Reiki weaken neither another person nor themselves. In fact, both people—the person giving the treatment and the one receiving it—will be charged with Reiki by the cosmos. If, during a Reiki session, you breathe as described in the following chapter about breathing, it will be impossible to draw energy out of a client.

19

When we want to express that a situation has triggered intensive feelings in our hearts or in the belly area, we say: "it touched me." We should feel lucky to have the possibility—because of the Reiki power—to learn the art of touching.

Touching and healing are two aspects of one unity. All human beings on our planet automatically touch the spot when they have bumped their heads. In many cultures, people shake hands, kiss, or embrace each other as a greeting. Through this first touch, a sensitive individual directly feels on which level the encounter with the other person will take place.

Animals are apparently similar to us in this respect: Tao, our cat, seems to know within seconds whether love, energy, fear, or indifference are coming from the hand that touches her.

Here is a simple partner exercise for this topic:
• Give your partner your hand or place it on an area of his/her body. Don't say whether you are letting love and caring flow into the touch, but let him/her feel what you are radiating. Change places and repeat this exercise as long as it's fun for the two of you.

The laying on of hands is one of the most natural things in the world. In Japan, it is called *Te a te*, and my father-in-law recently told me while we enjoyed a glass of sake that he always places his hands on the spot when he has pain. In Europe, this art was unfortunately lost after World War Two. My mother remembers that there was someone in her village who laid hands on the sick villagers.

Once again, women are somewhat ahead of us men in the art of touching. Because of their maternal instincts, their basic nature lets them be willing to touch others, as well as themselves, in a loving way and without any sexual* ulterior motives. Touching brings joy and well-being to the person who touches and the person who is touched.

There are actually just two types of touching, conscious and loving or unconscious, lukewarm touching. Back when I was a fresh-faced Reiki teacher, I told my students that they could treat themselves while watching television. Today, I see things differently and explain to the students: Be as collected and meditative as possible during a treatment without becoming tense. Give your patient—or yourself, if you are touching yourself—everything that you have. Let your entire heart, your entire being flow into the touch without holding anything back at all.

Imagine that this would be the last moment of your life.

A Reiki treatment done in such a way is pure meditation.

When you treat another person, be sure that you are open for everything that your senses encounter; however, don't let yourself be carried away by your senses, if at all possible. Be attentiveness personified: Register every thought, every feeling, every inspiration, even if it may appear to be completely irrelevant. Take an exact look at your patient. Observe the color of his/her skin and the position of the body. Are the limbs all stretched out evenly? Is the spinal column straight or does one of the vertebras stand out? Does the body move during the treatment? Does it twitch? Is it cold or warm, cool or hot? Is the respiration deep or shallow, even or uneven? Do you feel tension, stress, emotions, or anything else? What kind of facial expression does your client have? How does his/her aura radiate?

Remember all of this information, work with it, and—if you consider it relevant—tell it to your patient afterward. If you don't trust your memory, keep a pen and notepad ready.

So Chiryo
(treatment) builds upon Reiji
(devotion) and Gassho (medita-
tive posture/attitude). Only when
we can devote ourselves without be-
ing prejudiced by our thoughts and
feelings, will we become an instru-
ment for the universal life
energy.

But now we'll move on to the next important topic, which has often been neglected in Western Reiki up to now: breathing.

* Sexual feelings are the most natural in the world. However, if sexuality is suppressed, it appears again in another, often undesired, place. Up to now, only male students have asked me what they can do when they are sexually stimulated during a Reiki treatment. The simplest method is to think of something else! If the arousal is so strong that this method doesn't work, then inhale through your nose and imagine that the energy flows into your body through your first chakra. Just like the breath is drawn into the belly, the energy is drawn up in the opposite direction, through the chakras 1 through 6, to the nose. It briefly flows out of the body at that point, in order to flow back into the energy channel with exhalation and then descends into the first chakra. The energy again flows briefly out of the body there, and the whole process is repeated with the next breath.

The Breath

The bridge between the body and consciousness is the breath. In all esoteric traditions, there is knowledge of the special meaning of the breath.

Human beings and animals not only take in a mixture of various gases through respiration, but a mysterious something that we call Reiki in our circles. In India, it is called *Prana*, in China *Chi*, in Japan *Ki*, and Wilhelm Reich called it *orgon energy*.

My spiritual master Osho and my Tai Chi teacher Da Liu, from whom I was permitted to learn the fundamentals of Tai Chi during a six-month visit to New York in the mid-1980's, called the breath the vehicle. The energy that flows in with it is the actual passenger: the elixir of life.

In India and Egypt, for thousands of years there have been adepts who have themselves buried alive for a certain period of time. One of these people supposedly survived this exercise for twenty years. He had learned to absorb the life energy into his energy system in another way than through the breath in order to survive like this without oxygen. Every skin cell is capable of breathing and does this without our conscious mind.

There are also a group of people who have learned through practice to nourish themselves from *Prana* and only eat little or no "solid" food at all. I don't want to talk you into letting yourself be buried alive or giving up eating. I'm actually interested in something very simple and unspectacular: Learning to use the breath as a vehicle.

Joshin Kokyuu-Ho

For this purpose, Dr. Usui taught his students a breathing technique called *Joshin Kokyuu-Ho*. Translated into English, this means something like "the breathing method for cleansing the spirit." A variation of this technique is also used in Tai Chi and in other martial arts in order to learn to feel and intensify the flow of energy. We also use it to charge ourselves with energy.

According to Dr. Usui, it is done in the following manner:

• Sit down comfortably, keep your spine as straight as possible without becoming tense, and inhale slowly through your nose. Imagine that you are breathing in not only air through your nose but also the Reiki energy through your crown chakra. Many of you will directly feel how the energy enters through the crown chakra. I personally feel it to be a kind of ecstatic pressure or like something sweet that gently falls on me and energizes me. Other people may feel it to be light or warm. If you do not directly feel it, don't worry about it and continue to breathe calmly and serenely.

With time, the effect of this exercise and a strong feel of the energy flowing through you will make itself known. Feel how your entire body is enriched with energy during this kind of breathing and draw the breath far down into your belly, down to the energy center two or three fingerwidths beneath the navel. In Japan, this center is called *Tanden*, and the Chinese call it *Tantien*.

The Tanden

The *Tanden* is the center of the body, the seat of a person's vitality. As you will see below, the Tanden plays a leading role in Dr. Usui's hand positions.

Hold your breath and the energy you have drawn in with it in the Tanden for a few seconds. This is not a matter of getting into the *Guinness Book of Records*, so be loving and gentle with yourself in this exercise. We want to supply the body with love and energy, not stress and a fear of life. While holding your breath, imagine that the energy from the Tanden spreads throughout your entire body and energizes it.

Now exhale through your mouth. While doing this, imagine that the breath and the Reiki energy not only flow out of your mouth, but also from your fingertips and the tips of your toes and out of your hand and foot chakras. This is how we become a clear channel of Reiki. The energy flows into us from the cosmos and back again to the cosmos. The energy cycle from the macrocosm to the microcosm, and vice versa, has been completed.

In Tai Chi and Qigong, the following is always recommended for similar breathing exercises: Keep the tongue on the roof of your mouth, touching your front teeth while inhaling and then let it come down and rest on the bottom of the mouth while exhaling.

I prefer to show my students this exercise while standing since it's quite easy to feel the Tanden in the belly that way; when we experience it ourselves, we don't have to depend upon what other people say about it. We all have our energy centers in places that vary a bit from individual to individual.

Here is the exercise:

• Stand with both feet parallel to each other, the legs shoulderwidth apart. The tips of the feet point straight ahead. Now bend both knees a bit until you feel the central point beneath the navel in the Tanden. Hold this position and proceed as described above. Inhale and exhale deeply, evenly, and slowly for ten minutes. Feel how the breath and the energy flow through you as you do this.

Experiment with this technique while you treat yourself or others. I personally use it during almost all of the treatment. Chetna only uses it when she wants to provide specific areas of the body with additional energy.

As described in the next chapter, Dr. Usui employed not only the laying on of hands but also massage, pressure, and gentle tapping. So if you want to integrate acupressure with a Reiki treatment or charge specific acupuncture points and smaller areas of the body with Reiki, breathe as described above and very consciously give off the energy while exhaling. If you use pressure, increase it while exhaling and let go of it while inhaling.

Contraindication: Reiki practitioners who have very high blood pressure or asthma should not use this breathing technique. If you have a feeling of constriction, stop immediately. Inhale and exhale in a normal way by letting your breath follow its own course.

Storing Life Energy in the Tanden

Chetna has been experimenting with the healing methods of Haruchika Noguchi (1911-1976), one of the greatest healers in the history of Japan, since the mid-1980's. He gives the following instructions on storing the life energy in the Tanden in order to let it flow out of the hands:

"Calm your mind and your breathing so that the energy becomes pure (in my experience, our energy, our breath becomes impregnated by emotions and thoughts, which is why our first goal should be cleansing the energy and the breath). "Then inhale deeply from below through the spine and let the energy flow into the Tanden. Hold the breath there and with it the Tanden will be enriched with energy. Exhale through your fingers. As soon as you feel the energy flow into your fingers and the palms of your hands, begin the treatment."

Noguchi called his treatment technique *Yuki.* It is done in the following manner:

- Begin with the exercise above.
- Concentrate the energy in your hands, fold them (Gassho) and imagine that you are inhaling and exhaling through your folded hands. Deepen your breathing more and more so that you are apparently inhaling through your (folded) hands into the Tanden and exhaling in turn. While you touch an area of the body that is negatively charged, you will feel a tingling in your hands. Let your hands rest on this area of the body until the tingling has disappeared.

The Healing Techniques

Dr. Usui employed a series of healing techniques that he complied into a wonderful whole, the Usui Reiki Ryoho (system). In the interview already published in *Reiki, The Legacy of Dr. Usui*, Dr. Usui responded to the question of whether the *Usui Reiki Ryoho* uses medications and if there would be any type of side effects: "It uses neither medications nor instruments. It uses only looking, blowing, stroking, (light) tapping, and touching (of the afflicted part of the body). This is what heals diseases." Without these techniques, it would not be possible to understand the intuitive body work of Dr. Usui.

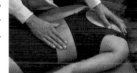

Touching (photo 1)

Massaging (photo 2)

1. He touched the diseased parts of the body.
2. He massaged them (photo 2)
3. He tapped* them (photo 3)
4. He stroked them (photo 4)
5. He blew on them (photo 5)
6. He fixed his gaze on them for two to three minutes (photo 6)
And there is an extra technique that I personally like very much:
7. He specifically gave them energy (photo 7)

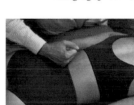

Tapping (photo 3)

One Japanese Reiki school teaches that Dr. Usui received the Reiki energy with his left hand and passed it on with his right hand. He is said to have brought the fingertips of his left hand together with the thumb, as if he were holding a raw egg. The fingertips of the middle finger and ring finger of the right hand are said to have touched the tip of the right thumb. The little finger and the index finger were said to have stood away from the middle and ring finger at a ninety-degree angle (photo 7).

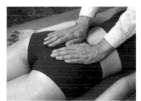

Stroking (photo 4)

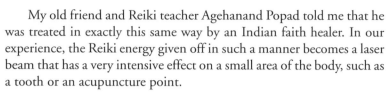

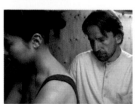

Blowing (photo 5)

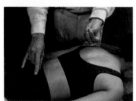

Looking (photo 6)

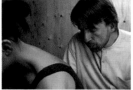

Specific direction of energy
(photo 7)

My old friend and Reiki teacher Agehanand Popad told me that he was treated in exactly this same way by an Indian faith healer. In our experience, the Reiki energy given off in such a manner becomes a laser beam that has a very intensive effect on a small area of the body, such as a tooth or an acupuncture point.

The distance-healing techniques that Dr. Usui used do not need to be mentioned in detail here. He supposedly used them often, even when the person to be treated was in the next room. He also recommended that we work with photographs whenever possible.

* *Da Liu* says that the tapping technique of Chen T'wan, a Taoist philosopher, was established in the Tenth Century. The traditional way of tapping was along the psychic channels—Tu Mo, Jen Mo, Tai Mo, Ch'ueng Mo, Yang Wei Mo, Yin Wei Mo, Yang Chiao, and Ying Chiao. (See the *Taoist Health Exercise Book* by Da Liu, Athena Books, ISBN 1-56924-901-6). In Japan, even your hairdresser can give you a percussion massage. For this purpose, either the palms of the hands or the three sides of the slightly closed fist (see photo 3) are used. Some martial-arts artists even require clubs, bricks, or knives for this purpose! Please don't try this!

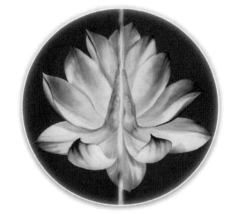

霊
氣

Reiki Ryoho Hikkei

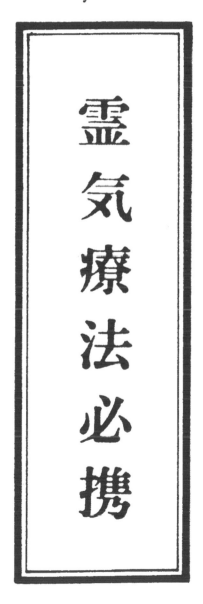

Reiki Ryoho Hikkei

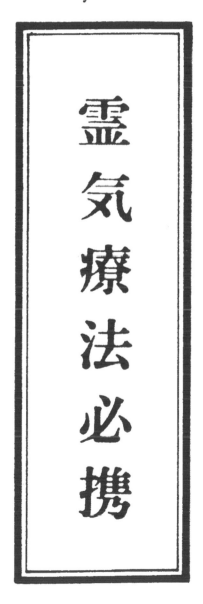

Dr. Usui's Hand Positions

The original hand positions of Dr. Usui are shown in the following. He divided them into eleven chapters. The Japanese terms, which I consider important, are set in italics. My notes and explanations are in parentheses. My wife Chetna and I translated them from the Japanese. Since Dr. Usui mainly, but not exclusively, used his right hand to treat people, we have taken the photos to reflect this. For some positions, related to very small areas of the body, I only used one, two, or three fingers. There is no deeper meaning in the choice of the fingers.

Whether left-handers should do the treatments with their dominant, left hand is not for me to decide. Please try it out on your own.

The body size of the patient and the size of your hands determine the exact location of the hand positions. If your hands are small or your patient is very large, you may possibly have to add an additional hand position here and there.

There are fundamentally no rules about the length of a treatment. In the case of pain, Dr. Usui recommends holding your hands on or over the affected area of the body until the pain has disappeared. Let your hands take their own course, no matter whether they want to stay for one, ten, or thirty minutes in one position. Mr. Ogawa recommended staying in the head positions for about thirty minutes. In my opinion, the most important thing in all of this is following your own intuition and your hands.

I consider it important before a specific treatment to explain to patients exactly what parts of the body will be touched so that they can be prepared for it. The more relaxed the patient is, the more pleasant the treatment will be. However, the Reiki energy even flows when patients are tense, comatose, or skeptical.

When you work with the *Reiji* method, you naturally won't know ahead of time to which areas of the body your hands will devote themselves. It is important for you to make it as easy as you can for your patient to trust you as much as possible.

So that you won't be overwhelmed by hundreds of photos, we have explained the treatments for certain body areas, as well as the most frequent health disorders and complaints with detailed illustrated hand positions (photos) in the first chapter. A few lines about the functions of the inner organs have also been added. Only the hand positions are shown for rare illnesses (as in Dr. Usui's *Original Reiki Handbook*). All of the hand positions from Dr. Usui's *Original Reiki Handbook* are reproduced in photos at the end of this book in the order of their appearance. You can look up the exact positions in all of the special cases here.

I don't know whether or not left-handers should practice with their left, dominant hand. Just try it out youself!

On pages 72-76 you can find the exact positions for all special ailments.

The way to find the exact positions of the vertebrae is described in detail (and illustrated) on page 79.

Index of the Reiki Ryoho Hikkei

目次 1)

一、臼井霊気療法教義 2)

二、公開伝授説明 3)

三、療法指針 4)

四、明治天皇御製 5)

29

The Reiki-Ryoho-Handbook

Page 20 of the original book is reproduced here. It describes some of Dr. Usui's treatment positions.

心　　　肺咽舌口　耳　　鼻

臓　　　　喉

霊気療法必携

鼻骨、鼻翼、眉間、頸部（第

一、二、三、頸椎）

耳孔、耳ノ前部及後部（乳嘴

突起）第一頸椎

唇ヲ除ケテ手ニテ蔽フ

舌ノ上面、舌根

甲状軟骨、頸部

肺部、背部肩胛骨ノ内側、第

二、三、四、五、六胸椎

心臓部、第五、六、七、頸椎、第一

–1–
Basic Treatment for Specific Parts of the Body

Forehead, temples, back of the head, throat/back of the neck, on the head, stomach, and intestines.

(The Chinese characters for the back of the neck and throat are identical. Consequently, it is unclear which part of the body is meant. The best approach is to cover both the back of the neck and the throat. Since most problems that we have take place in our minds, Dr. Usui also recommends treating the head directly. This isn't just a matter of treating injuries but also relaxing psychological tensions and energetic barriers. There is a wonderful Hindu meditation that teaches us to gently lay the palms of the hands on the cheekbones and, keeping our hands as light as a feather, touch our eyeballs. With this very light touch, we can put ourselves into a deep state of meditation within a few minutes. When doing this, let the Reiki energy—and the symbols, if you have learned them—flow.)

The Head:

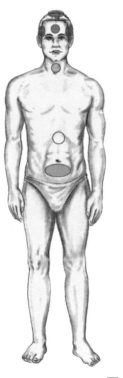

1 Forehead

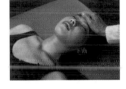

2 Temples

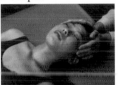

3 Back of head

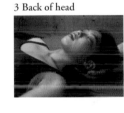

4 Back of neck

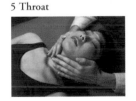

5 Throat

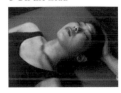

6 On the head

7 Stomach and intestines

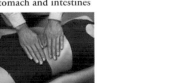
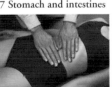

Forehead ▪
Temples ▪
Back of head ▪
Back of neck ▪
Throat ▪
On the head ▪
Stomach and intestines ▪ ▫

The Technique for Lowering Fever, Genetsu-Ho:

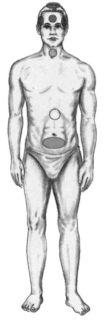

The same hand positions as for the head and *Byogen Chiryo* (treatment of the source of an illness).

(The two above-mentioned techniques are not explained in detail. For the *Genetsu-Ho* technique, Mr. Ogawa recommends letting the hand or hands rest on the head in particular.

I have personally determined that fever can have a healing effect, as long as it doesn't get too high—less than 39.5 degrees C (103 degrees F). In this case, I leave it up to my intuition to decide whether I should try to bring the fever down or not. If the fever is higher, I would in any case use the methods suggested by Dr. Usui before or while bringing the person to a member of the medical profession for monitoring.

In a natural way, a moderate fever detoxifies a body that has experienced an increase in toxins. Afterward, a spinal column that has lost its equilibrium may possibly even straighten up on its own.)

1 Forehead

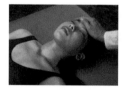

2 Temples

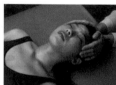

3 Back of head

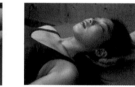

4 Back of neck

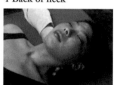

5 Throat

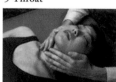

6 On the head

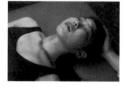

7 Stomach and intestines

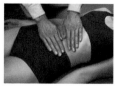

■ *Forehead*

■ *Temples*

■ *Back of head*

■ *Back of neck*

■ *Throat*

■ *On the head*

■ □ *Stomach and intestines*

32

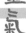

The Eyes:

The eyes, the point between the eyes and nose, between the eyes and the temples; the first, second, and third cervical vertebrae.

(Our eyes are constantly strained in a world and economy based on visual stimuli. The biggest malefactors are watching television too long, concentrated reading, and work at the computer. An effective remedy for this is filling a little pillow with flaxseed, which can be charged beforehand with Reiki One or Two.

Otherwise, remember to follow the rule of taking a break at least once every hour; also, turn away from your monitor/book frequently and look at an object that is five or six yards away from you.

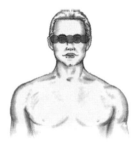

8 Eyes

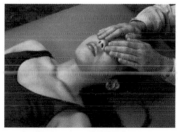

9 Between eyes and nose

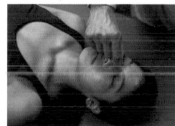

10 Between eyes and temples

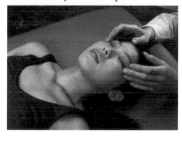

43 Cervical vertebrae area 1-3

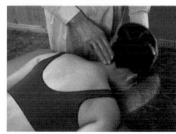

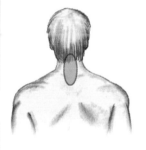

Eyes ■

Between eyes and nose ■

Between eyes and temples ■

Cervical vertebrae area 1-3 ■

33

The Nose:

Nasal bone, side of the nose, middle of forehead, throat/back of neck, cervical vertebrae area 1-3

(Nose and sinus complaints, as well as allergies, are increasing rapidly in our polluted environment. Fortunately, through a special diet we can avoid the worst problems related to the above conditions: In any case, avoid all milk products and mucous-producing foods, at least as long as the complaints persist.

A good home remedy for cleansing the nose is one teaspoon of freshly grated horseradish added to a cup of boiling water. Drink like tea.)

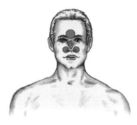

■ *Nasal bone*
■ *Side of the nose*
■ *Middle of forehead*

11 Nasal bone

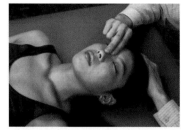

12 Side of the nose

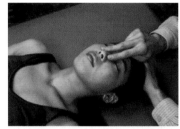

13 Middle of forehead

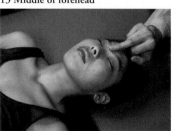

4 Back of neck

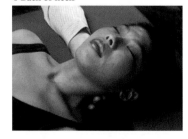

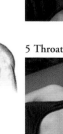

■ *Back of neck*
■ *Throat*
■ *Cervical vertebrae area*

5 Throat

43 Cervical vertebrae area 1-3

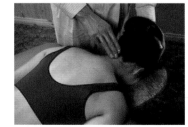

The Ears:

The ear canal, in front of the ear—behind the ear—the protruding cartilage in the auricle (these three are shown in a photo), the first cervical vertebra.

(If you treat both ears at the same time, there is also a bonus effect: The two brain hemispheres are synchronized. In our experience, hands resting on the ears may possibly raise up an inch or so from the body. They stay there for a while and then perhaps move even further from the body and work in the aura before they rest on the physical body again.

I also treat clients who have had slight strokes in this manner. Afterward, you can "park" your hands on the *Tanden* for ten or fifteen minutes.)

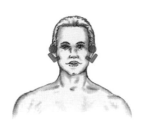

Ear canal ■

In front of the ear ■
behind the ear

14 Auditory canal entering

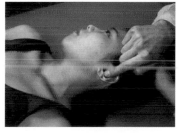

15 In front of and behind the ear

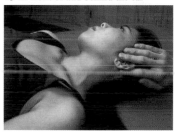

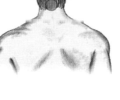

42 Cervical vertebrae area 1

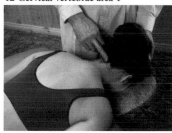

In front of the ear ■
behind the ear

Cervical vertebrae 1 ■

The Mouth:

Place the hand over the mouth without closing off the lips.

(Test for yourself how this feels when you cover and close off the mouth—and then you will know why Dr. Usui says we shouldn't do this. But keeping our mouths closed once in a while can certainly be a good exercise for many people! As in English, there is a Japanese saying *chinmoku wa kin*: "silence is golden."

However, if a patient is too still—in the sense of becoming unconscious—there is a highly effective accupressure point at the center of the upper lip (see photo 21) that can bring the person back to consciousness.)

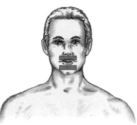

■ *Over the mouth
(don't close the lips)*

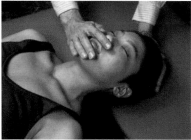

16 Over the mouth without closing off lips.
(I put my left hand on my crown chakra in this
position because it feels right to me.)

(21 In the middle of the upper lip)

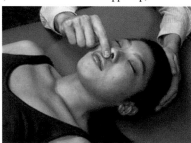

The Tongue:

On the tongue, on the root of the tongue.

(This hand position may be unpleasant for some people; because of hygienic reasons and because it reminds us of the commonly feared visit to the dentist. Consequently, it is perhaps better to treat the tongue with distance Reiki. If you can't do this or you consider a direct treatment to be more effective, put on a fresh pair of latex gloves. Translator's note: be sure neither of you have an allergy to Latex!
A TIP FOR MEDITATION: I read in a book about the Indian saint Ramakrishna that he had his wife write holy symbols on his tongue. So I asked my wife to also do this for me. Although I had to laugh at first because it tickled, the Reiki symbols melted in my mouth, so to speak. It was a wonderful feeling.)

17 On the tongue (wear latex gloves)

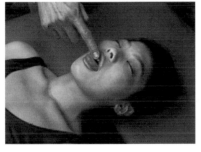

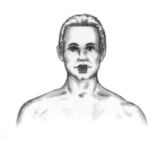

On the tongue ■
Root of the tongue ■

18 On the root of the tongue (wear latex gloves)

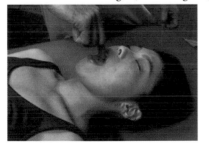

The Throat:

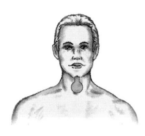

The cartilage in the throat (Adam's apple), the throat/back of neck.

(From an anatomical perspective, the throat is a very easily injured part of the body. Because of this, we quickly feel ourselves threatened when someone encircles our throat. So please be especially sensitive and gentle in this position. I personally prefer the illustrated position, but there are also other possibilities. You can, for example, lean both hands on your client's lower jaw while standing or sitting behind him/her. This will allow your hands to rest an inch or so above the throat.

SOME MORE TIPS: I recommend ginger tea against sore throat complaints. Grate a teaspoon-sized piece of ginger into a cup and fill the cup with boiling water. Let it cool a bit, then try drinking it. If you tolerate a stronger mixture, grate some more ginger into it. Drink this tea in small sips. Zinc lozenges are also very effective against a sore throat.)

■ *Cartilage in throat*

■ *Throat/back of neck*

19 Cartilage in throat

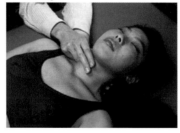

4 Back of neck

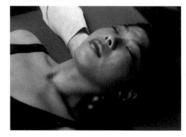

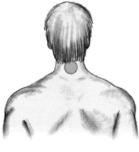

5 Throat

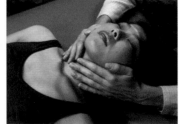

■ *Throat/back of neck*

The Lungs:

The lung area, between the shoulder blades, the second—sixth thoracic vertebrae.

(The lungs provide our body with vital oxygen, of which one-fifth of the air that we inhale is composed. With the help of this oxygen, our body cells burn sugar. This produces energy. Carbon dioxide is also expelled through the lungs.

As described in the chapter about breathing, Dr. Usui was quite meticulous in teaching his students what it means to inhale deeply into the *Tanden*.

But even when we breathe normally, meaning without consciously drawing in energy from the cosmos, it is helpful to breathe into the belly. If this is difficult for you at the beginning, it may be helpful to place one or both hands on the belly and then draw the air in to that point. Our experience has shown that abdominal breathing can be learned within a short amount of time.)

22 Lungs

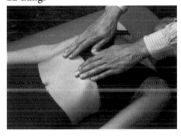

44 Between the shoulder blades

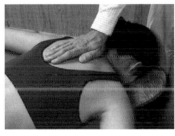

Lung area

45 Thoracic vertebrae area 2-6

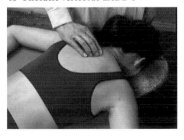

Between the shoulder blades

Thoracic vertebrae 2-6

The Heart;

The heart area, cervical vertebrae 5-7, 45 thoracic vertebrae area 1-5.

(As we all know, the heart pumps our blood through the aorta, the main artery, and from there through the remaining arteries to our organs and into the tissue. The blood provides both with nutrients and oxygen. As soon as it has delivered the oxygen, it is guided through the veins to the lungs. Here it is once again enriched with oxygen. From the lungs, the blood flows back to the heart and the cycle begins anew.

The heart also plays a leading role in our energy body. In the heart chakra, the coarser energies from the lower chakras and the subtle energies from the upper chakras are changed into usable healing energies. Then these flow through our arms into our hands.

A Reiki treatment of the heart calms and helps the client to feel loved and protected.)

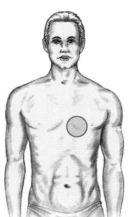

□ *Heart area*

23 Heart

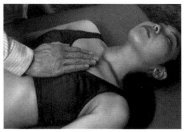

46 Cervical vertebrae area 5-7

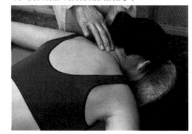

47 Thoracic vertebrae area 1-5

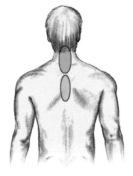

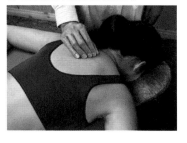

■ *Cervical vertebrae 5-7*

□ *Thoracic vertebrae 1-5*

40

The liver area, thoracic vertebrae 8-10, especially on the right side of the body.

(The liver is the largest inner organ in our body, and there is a reason for this: Its main task is to detoxify the toxins and waste products and produce or process new chemicals. So be nice to your liver and don't make its life—and yours—too difficult.

In case of liver damage, you should avoid fatty foods, consumption of alcohol, nicotine, and medications. Fortunately, the liver is capable of regenerating itself; however, this doesn't happen overnight. A liver that has been severely damaged by drug abuse or jaundice needs months, if not years, to recover its health again.

So treat the liver over a longer period of time in keeping with the severity of the health disorder. I suggest at least one-half hour for the manner of treatment recommended by Dr. Usui.)

The Liver:

肝
臟

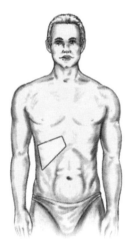

24 Liver

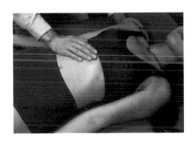

45 Thoracic vertebrae area 8-10
(mainly on the right side)

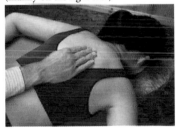

Liver ☐

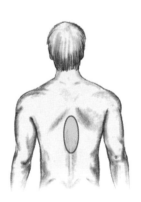

Thoracic vertebrae 8-10 ▨
(especially on right side)

41

The Stomach:

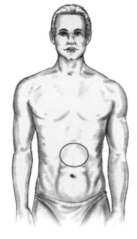

The stomach area, thoracic vertebrae 4 and 6-10.

(The stomach serves as a reservoir for the food that we eat, as well as the starting place for the digestion. This is where the digestive juices are mixed with the food. These juices turn the food into a mush, which is then pressed through the duodenum into the intestines below.

However, the stomach is also the seat of our emotions. There is definitely a reason for saying "I can't stomach this" or "I have to first digest that."

In emotional crises—including when children cry, I suggest resting both hands on the stomach and intestines for at least fifteen minutes. I personally always treat the stomach and intestines at the same time; but it is also possible to treat them separately.)

☐ *Stomach*

7 Stomach and intestines

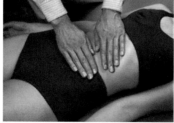

49 Thoracic vertebrae area 4 and 6-10

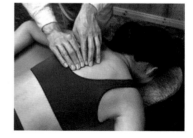

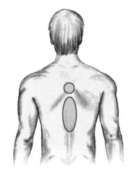

▢ *Thoracic vertebra 4*

▢ *Thoracic vertebrae 6-10*

The Intestines:

腸

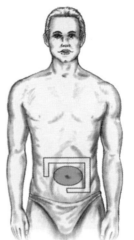

The upper and lower sides of the large intestine, the area of the small intestine (around the navel), the thoracic vertebrae 6-10, the lumbar vertebrae 2-5, the buttocks.

(From the duodenum, the mush that has been pressed out of the stomach reaches the attached small intestine. This is where digestion actually takes place. From here, the mush moves on to the large intestine. During this journey, nutrients and water are removed from the mush.

Since the intestines have many curves and bends, it can easily happen that harmful substances deposited in these curves and bends are not eliminated during the digestive process.

Consequently, we must be very conscientious in treating the intestines. The treatment of the intestines helps remove these toxins from the intestinal walls so that they can be eliminated. Other methods of getting rid of these substances are enemas, fasting cures, or taking certain healing herbs. However, this should only be done according to a doctor's instructions.)

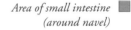

Upper and lower side of ☐
large intestine

Area of small intestine ■
(around navel)

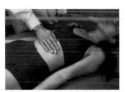

25 Large intestine—upper

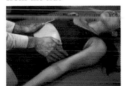

26 Large intestine—lower
from the side

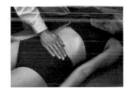

27 Area of small intestine

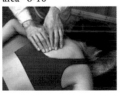

49 Thoracic vertebrae
area* 6-10

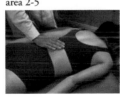

68 Lumbar vertebrae
area 2-5

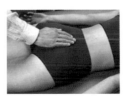

54 Sacrum, coccyx

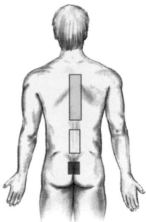

* Note on photo 49: in this position, you could also place a hand between the shoulder blades—somewhat lower than in photo 44 (p. 75)

Thoracic vertebrae 6-10 ■

Lumbar vertebrae 2-5 ☐ ■

Buttocks ■

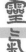

The Bladder:

膀
胱

The bladder area, lumbar vertebrae 4-5

(The bladder is filled by a constantly dripping flow of urine from the kidneys through the ureter. The urine is then eliminated through the urethra. A woman's urethra is very short and unprotected because of its anatomic position. This is why women often must battle urogenital inflammations. For treatment, let your hands rest on the bladder and somewhat below it for at least fifteen minutes.

Because of anatomic reasons, the danger of inflammation is not very great for men. However, they have another vulnerable point: the prostate gland, which lies directly beneath the bladder and through which the urethra passes. When the prostate gland is swollen, there is difficulty in urination. Treat the lower bladder area for at least fifteen minutes.)

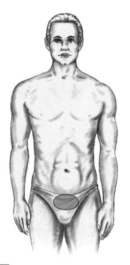

28 Bladder area

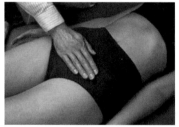

78 Lumbar vertebrae area 4-5

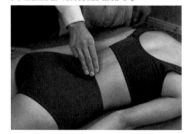

■ *Bladder*

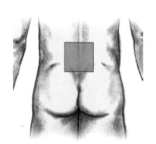

■ *Lumbar vertebrae 4-5*

44

The Uterus:

The area of the uterus, both sides of the uterus, the thoracic vertebrae 9-12, the lumbar vertebrae 1-5, the sacrum, the coccyx.

(The uterus is the part of the body—like the cosmos—that is the first stage in our process of becoming a human being. We don't arrive on the earth as complete human beings—we must first achieve this state! With this aspect in mind, it is very important to treat the uterus with extra special attention, even when there isn't a future citizen of the earth living in it at the moment.)

29 Uterus area

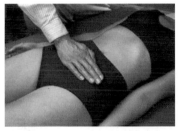

30 Uterus on both sides, ovaries

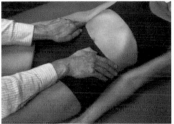

Uterus area ■
Both sides of uterus ■

52 Thoracic vertebrae area 9-12

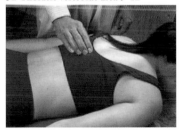

58 Lumbar vertebrae area 1-5

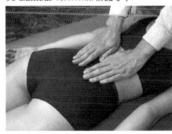

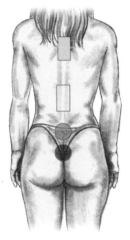

54 Sacrum, coccyx

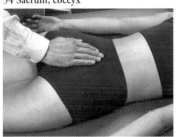

Thoracic vertebrae 9-12 ■
Lumbar vertebrae 1-5 □ ■
Sacrum ■
Coccyx ■

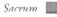

45

The Kidneys:

腎

臟

The kidney area, thoracic vertebrae 11-12

(The kidneys filter about 130 milliliters of our blood per minute. This results in about 1200 liters per day! The waste products found in the blood are diverted from the kidneys as urine and then eliminated from the body in this manner. I treat the kidneys for at least fifteen minutes when there has been any kind of poisoning of the system, as well as for shock, subnormal temperatures, and hypothermia of the kidneys.

In our experience, the client begins to breathe more deeply as soon as the hands are laid on his/her kidneys.)

55 Kidney area

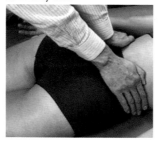

56 Thoracic vertebrae area 11-12

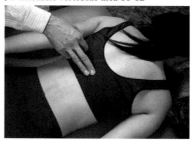

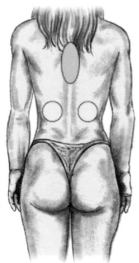

■ *Thoracic vertebrae 11-12*

□ *Kidney area*

Treatment of Half of the Body,
Hanshin Chiryo:

The muscles, the tendons of the back of the neck, the shoulders, the spinal column, both sides of the spinal column, the hips, the buttocks. (Rub the spinal column on both sides from the buttocks to the medulla oblongata.)

(This method brings a client who is poorly grounded or put into a trance-like state by the treatment back down to earth. I therefore recommend using this technique, except for the symptoms described by Dr. Usui, at the close of a treatment as well. Afterward, the client is quickly capable of getting up from the massage table in a refreshed and lively manner.)

57 Healing technique Hanshin Chiryo 1

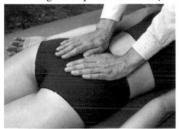

58 Healing technique Hanshin Chiryo 2

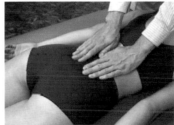

59 Healing technique Hanshin Chiryo 3

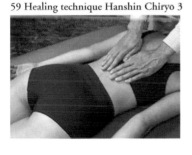

60 Healing technique Hanshin Chiryo 4

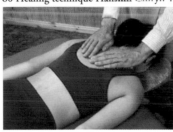

61 Healing technique Hanshin Chiryo 5

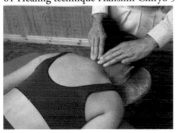

Hanshin Chiryo

Rub along both sides of the spinal column, from the buttocks to the medulla oblongata

47

Treatment of Abdomen, Chiryo-Gedoku-Ho (Detoxification Technique):

(These two techniques are not explained in detail. However, Mr. Ogawa told us how they are applied.

Tanden Chiryo: Place one hand on the Tanden and the other on the back behind it.

Gedoku-Ho: Rest your hand in the *Tanden-Chiryo* position for thirteen minutes and imagine that all of the toxins are leaving the body. This technique has proved to be very successful against constipation and the consequences of excessive use of medication. The client's stomach frequently begins to rumble after a few minutes of the treatment, so please tell your clients in advance that they shouldn't feel ashamed because of this. Here in Japan, rumbling of the stomach and other bodily noises are something very private and people try to suppress them in any case!)

Tanden Chiryo

Place one hand on the Tanden and one hand on the back behind it.

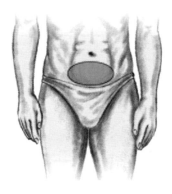

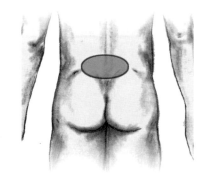

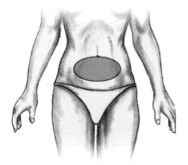

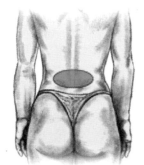

– 2 –
Functional Disorders of the Nerves

You will find the corresponding photos on pages 72-77.

(The head area is always treated in the following positions. Follow your intuition and possibly treat the throat/back of the neck area as well.)

Neurasthenia (nervous debility):

The head area, the eyes, the heart, the stomach and intestines, the genital organs, treatment of the area where the illness originated (*Byogen Chiryo*), treatment of the half of the body (*Hanshin Chiryo*, see p. 47).

Photos: 1 Forehead, 2 Temples, 3 Back of head, 6 On the head, 8 Eyes, 23 Heart, 7 Stomach and intestines, 32 Genital organs, 57 Healing technique Hanshin Chiryo 1, 58 Healing technique Hanshin Chiryo 2, 59 Healing technique Hanshin Chiryo 3, 60 Healing technique Hanshin Chiryo 4, 61 Healing technique Hanshin Chiryo 5

Hysteria:

As above

Photos: 1 Forehead, 2 Temples, 3 Back of head, 6 On the head, 8 Eyes, 23 Heart, 7 Stomach and intestines, 32 Genital organs, 57 Healing technique Hanshin Chiryo 1, 58 Healing technique Hanshin Chiryo 2, 59 Healing technique Hanshin Chiryo 3, 60 Healing technique Hanshin Chiryo 4, 61 Healing technique Hanshin Chiryo 5

Cerebral Anemia :

The head area, stomach and intestines, the heart.

Photos: 1 Forehead, 2 Temples, 3 Back of head, 6 On the head, 7 Stomach and intestines, 23 Heart

Cerebral Hyperanemia (Vascular Congestion in the Brain):

As above

Photos: 1 Forehead, 2 Temples, 3 Back of head, 6 On the head, 7 Stomach and intestines, 23 Heart

Meningitis:

As above

Photos: 1 Forehead, 2 Temples, 3 Back of head, 6 On the head, 7 Stomach and intestines, 23 Heart

Encephalitis: As above

Photos: 1 Forehead, 2 Temples, 3 Back of head, 6 On the head, 7 Stomach and intestines, 23 Heart

Headache: The head area—mainly the temples.

(Follow Dr. Usui's treatment tips by resting your hands on the head until the pain is gone. If you have learned Second Degree Reiki, use the power symbol as well.

Headaches can have many different causes. Frequently, the cause is simply dehydration: Immediately drink one or two glasses of water. The caffeine in a cup of coffee can also work wonders.

When the pain comes from the neck: Lay down on your bed so that your head hangs down from the edge of the bed. Relax for a few minutes.

Headaches often are often caused by chronically bad posture. In this case, I recommend the following book: *Pain Free, A Revolutionary Method for Stopping Chronic Pain* by Peter Egoscue, Bantam Doubleday Dell Pub. ISBN 0553106309. The title doesn't exaggerate!)

Photos: 2 Temples, 1 Forehead, 3 Back of head, 6 On the head

Insomnia: The head area—mainly the back of the head.

(Here we recommend a chakra hand position while falling asleep: Place one hand on the second chakra and the other hand on the fourth chakra. You can also suggest repose and falling asleep quickly to yourself by using the Reiki Two symbols. Think of a positive affirmation in your own words to help you fall asleep.

Learning Autogenic Training is also worthwhile.

However, the above tips are solely directed against the symptoms. Insomnia is usually related to psychological tensions and it is important to go directly to the roots of the problem. Find out where these tensions come from and try to resolve them.

One of my methods of meditation, which has already been printed elsewhere, recommends letting the entire day pass backward through your mind's eye—like rewinding a videotape. This will let you quickly work through things that haven't been digested yet.

Photos: 1 Forehead, 2 Temples, 3 Back of head, 6 On the head

Equilibrium Disorders, Dizziness: The head area—mainly the forehead.

Photos: 1 Forehead, 2 Temples, 3 Back of head, 6 On the head

Cerebral Hemorrhage:

Mainly the affected side, the heart, the stomach and intestines, the kidneys, and the paralyzed area.

Photos: 23 Heart, 7 Stomach and intestines, 55 kidney area

Epilepsy:

The head area*, the stomach and intestines.

(* In our experience, the head of an epileptic is too sensitive to touch. In this case, I treat the solar plexus and the *Tanden*.

During an epileptic seizure, the most important thing is to help the patient into a position where he/she cannot hurt himself/herself.)

Photos: 1 Forehead, 2 Temples, 3 Back of head, 6 On the head, 7 Stomach and intestines

St. Vitus's Dance:

The head area, the heart, the affected area(s) of the body, the palms of the hands, the soles of the feet, the half of the body (*Hanshin Chiryo*).

Photos: 1 Forehead, 2 Temples, 3 Back of head, 6 On the head, 23 Heart, 65 Palms of the hands, 66 Soles of the feet, 57 Healing technique Hanshin Chiryo 1, 58 Healing technique Hanshin Chiryo 2, 59 Healing technique Hanshin Chiryo 3, 60 Healing technique Hanshin Chiryo 4, 61 Healing technique Hanshin Chiryo 5

Basedow's Diesease

The head area, the eyes, the thyroid gland, the heart, the uterus, the half of the body (Hanshin Chiryo)

Photos: 1 Forehead, 2 Temples, 3 Back of head, 5 Throat (also covering the thyroid gland), 6 On the head, 23 Heart, 29 Area of uterus, 57 Healing technique Hanshin Chiryo 1, 58 Healing technique Hanshin Chiryo 2, 59 Healing technique Hanshin Chiryo 3, 60 Healing technique Hanshin Chiryo 4, 61 Healing technique Hanshin Chiryo 5

Neuralgia (Nerve Pain), Paralysis:

The head area, stomach and intestines in order to regulate the bowel movement, the affected area(s) of the body.

Photos: 1 Forehead, 2 Temples, 3 Back of head, 6 On the head, 7 Stomach and intestines

51

Hiccups: The diaphragm, the forehead, cervical vertebrae 3-5
(We use the power symbol for hiccups, just as we do for pain. If possible, trace it onto the diaphragm, the forehead, and the cervical vertebrae 3-5. If this isn't possible, either project the symbol onto the respective parts of the body with your eyes or let it flow out of your hands.)
Photos: 33 Diaphragm, 1 Forehead, 62 Cervical Vertebrae area 3-5

Aphasia
(Speech Disorders):   The forehead, the temples—mainly the left side, the throat area.
Photos: 1 Forehead, 2 Temples, 5 Throat

Writer's Cramp: The head area, the elbows, the thumbs.
(I encircle the thumb in my relaxed but clenched fist.)
Photos: 1 Forehead, 2 Temples, 3 Back of head, 6 On the head, 63 Elbows, 64 Thumbs

Tinnitus (Ringing in
the Ears):   The ears, the head area.
Photos: 14 Ear canal, 15 In front of and behind the ear, 1 Forehead, 2 Temples, 3 Back of head, 6 On the head

– 3 –
Functional Disorders of the Respiratory Organs (and Air Passages)

Inflammation of the Trachea (Windpipe)—
Bronchitis: The windpipe, the bronchial tubes.
Photos: 34 Windpipe, 35 Bronchial tubes

Coughing: The throat, the chest area, the affected area(s) of the body.
(We also use the power-intensification symbol for coughing. If you have learned Second Degree Reiki, draw the power symbol on a piece of material made of natural fibers and stick it onto your chest overnight. Avoid all mucous-producing foods for a week and eat much freshly grated ginger. Drink ginger tea with honey.)
Photos: 5 Throat, 22 Lungs—also cover the chest area

Asthma:

The head area, the chest area, beneath the sternum (the indentation beneath the sternum), the throat, the nose, the heart.

(A recipe, which I learned from my brother, helps against asthma: Grate 50 grams (1.6 ounces) of fresh horseradish and mix it with the juice of three large (organically grown) lemons and 500 grams (16 ounces) of organic honey. Take one tablespoon of this mixture before or after each meal for at least six weeks. Store the mixture in the refrigerator.

> Photos: 1 Forehead, 2 Temples, 3 Back of head, 6 On the head, 22 Lungs—also cover chest area, 37 Beneath the sternum, 5 Throat, 11 Nasal bone, 12 Sides of the nose, 23 Heart

Tuberculosis in the Lungs:

The head area, the affected part of the lungs, the stomach and intestines, the heart, the *Tanden.*

> Photos: 1 Forehead, 2 Temples, 3 Back of head, 6 On the head, 22 Lungs, 7 Stomach and intestines, 23 Heart, 31 Tanden

Pleurisy:

The head area, the affected area(s) of the body, the stomach and intestines, the *Tanden.*

> Photos: 1 Forehead, 2 Temples, 3 Back of head, 6 On the head, 7 Stomach and intestines, 31 Tanden

Pneumonia:

The head area, the heart, the affected body area(s), the *Tanden.*

> Photos: 1 Forehead, 2 Temples, 3 Back of head, 6 On the head, 23 Heart, 31 Tanden

Bronchial Hemorrhage (Blood-Spitting):

The lungs, the affected area of the body.

(This is a potentially fatal bleeding that is caused by the hollowing of small lung arteries.

> Photo: 22 Lungs

Nosebleed:

The nose.

(A pillow under the back of the neck and treating the first five cervical vertebrae does wonders. A pressure massage of the medulla oblongata shows good results. The patient's head should be leaned back when doing this.)

> Photos: 11 Nasal bone, 12 Sides of the nose

53

Emphyema (Pleurisy with
Formation of Pus):   The nose, middle of the forehead—or the point in the middle of the upper lip directly under the nose (the *Kanji* is not clear here; treat both in case of doubt).

> Photos: 11 Nasal bone, 12 Sides of the nose, 20 Middle of forehead, 21 Middle of upper lip

–––––––––––––––––––––––––––––––––––––

– 4 –
Functional Disorders of the Digestive Organs

Diseases
of the Esophagus: The esophagus, beneath the sternum, the stomach and intestines.

> Photos: 34 Windpipe, Esophagus, 37 Beneath the sternum, 7 Stomach and intestines

Gastritis, Gastric Ulcers, Stomach Cancer,
Gastralgia (Pain in the Stomach),
Gastroptosis,
Gastrectasis: The head area, beneath the sternum, the stomach and intestines.

> Photos: 1 Forehead, 2 Temples, 3 Back of head, 6 On the head, 37 Beneath the sternum, 7 Stomach and intestines

Enteritis, Intestinal Ulcers, Diarrhea,
Constipation, etc.:   The stomach and intestines.

> Photo: 7 Stomach and intestines

Appendicitis: The affected body area—mainly to the right next to the navel, the head area, the stomach and intestines.

> Photos: 38 Appendix, 1 Forehead, 2 Temples, 3 Back of head, 6 On the head, 7 Stomach and intestines

Intestinal Parasites: The head area, the stomach and intestines.

> Photos: 1 Forehead, 2 Temples, 3 Back of head, 6 On the head, 7 Stomach and intestines

(Wormwood drops, wormwood/clove/walnut tincture have already proved effective in driving some parasites from the intestines! Don't think that intestinal parasites only infest people in developing countries. Get advice from an expert naturopath.)

Hemorrhoids:

The anal area.
  Photo: 67 The anal area

Ascites in the Belly (Hydroperitoneum):

The head area, the abdominal area.
  (If possible, treat during the waning moon.)
    Photos: 1 Forehead, 2 Temples, 3 Back of head, 6 On the head,
    7 Stomach and intestines

Peritonitis (Inflammation of the Peritoneum):

The head area, the affected body area(s), the *Tanden*.
  Photos: 1 Forehead, 2 Temples, 3 Back of head, 6 On the head,
  31 Tanden

Hepatitis (Jaundice):

The head area, the stomach and intestines, the liver, the heart.
  (Caution: There are many types of jaundice that can only be diag-
nosed with certainty by a lab. Hepatitis A and E (which can only be
precisely determined by a lab by using a blood-count test) are extremely
contagious during the incubation period and should only be treated in
a hospital. After having jaundice, avoid fatty foods, alcohol, nicotine,
and, if possible, every type of medication for at least six months. After
consulting with your physician, have your blood values tested at regular
intervals.
    Photos: 1 Forehead, 2 Temples, 3 Back of head, 6 On the head,
    7 Stomach and intestines, 24 Liver, 23 Heart

Gallstones:

The liver, the affected body area(s), the stomach and intestines.
  Photos: 24 Liver, 7 Stomach and intestines

Inguinal Hernia:

The affected protruding body area(s), the abdomen (genital organs).
  Photo: 32 Genital organs

– 5 –
Functional Disorders of the Circulatory (Cardiovascular) System

(A tip from my spiritual master Osho: If you have heart problems, pay more attention to your outbreath. Exhale consciously and deeply and let the inbreath flowing in penetrate you, as if on its own.)

Inflammation of the Myocardium (Heart Muscle), Myocarditis: The head area, the heart, the liver, the kidneys, the bladder.
   (This condition can lead to cardiac failure in young people who are otherwise healthy.)
      Photos: 1 Forehead, 2 Temples, 3 Back of head, 6 On the head, 23 Heart, 24 Liver, 55 Kidney area, 28 Bladder area

Inflammation of the Membranes in the Heart: The heart.
      Photo: 23 Heart

Edema, Dropsy: The heart, the liver, the kidneys, the bladder.
   (If possible, treat during waning moon.)
      Photos: 23 Heart, 24 Liver, 55 Kidney area, 28 Bladder area

Arteriosclerosis (Arterial Calcification):   The head area, the heart, the kidneys, the stomach and intestines, the *Tanden.*
   (Eating a strict vegetarian diet—at least for a time without milk products—can counteract the calcification of arteries and high blood pressure. Even in an advanced stage, these conditions can often be completely reversed.)
      Photos: 1 Forehead, 2 Temples, 3 Back of head, 6 On the head, 23 Heart, 55 Kidney area, 7 Stomach and intestines, 31 Tanden

Chronic High Blood Pressure: As above.
      Photos: 1 Forehead, 2 Temples, 3 Back of head, 6 On the head, 23 Heart, 55 Kidney area, 7 Stomach and intestines, 31 Tanden

The head area, the heart, the stomach and intestines, affected body area(s).

Angina Pectoris:

> Photos: 1 Forehead, 2 Temples, 3 Back of head, 6 On the head, 23 Heart, 7 Stomach and intestines

Beriberi and Cardiac Failure Resulting from Beriberi:

The heart, the stomach and intestines, the affected leg(s).

> (Beriberi is a heart disorder based on a vitamin B1-thiamin-deficiency.)
> Photos: 23 Heart, 7 Stomach and intestines

– 6 –
Functional Disorders of the Metabolism and the Blood

Treatment for the origin of a disease *(Byogen Chiryo)*, the head, the heart, the stomach and intestines, the half of the body *(Hanshin Chiryo)*.

Anemia:

> Photos: 1 Forehead, 2 Temples, 3 Back of head, 4 Back of neck, 5 Throat, 6 On the head, 23 Heart, 7 Stomach and intestines, 57 Healing technique Hanshin Chiryo 1, 58 Healing technique Hanshin Chiryo 2, 59 Healing technique Hanshin Chiryo 3, 60 Healing technique Hanshin Chiryo 4, 61 Healing technique Hanshin Chiryo 5

Purpura (Diffuse Bleeding in the Skin's Surface at a Diameter of about 1/2 Inch):

The head area, the heart, the kidneys, the stomach and intestines, the body areas covered with lilac spots, the *Tanden*.

> Photos: 1 Forehead, 2 Temples, 3 Back of head, 6 On the head, 23 Heart, 55 Kidney area, 7 Stomach and intestines, 31 Tanden.

Scurvy: The head area, the lung area, the heart, the kidneys, the stomach and intestines, the half of the body (Hanshin Chiryo), the *Tanden.*

> Photos: 1 Forehead, 2 Temples, 3 Back of head, 6 On the head, 22 Lungs, 23 Heart, 55 Kidney area, 7 Stomach and intestines, 57 Healing technique Hanshin Chiryo 1, 58 Healing technique Hanshin Chiryo 2, 59 Healing technique Hanshin Chiryo 3, 60 Healing technique Hanshin Chiryo 4, 61 Healing technique Hanshin Chiryo 5, 31 Tanden

Diabetes: The head area, the heart, the liver, the pancreas, the stomach and intestines, the kidneys, the bladder, the half of the body *(Hanshin Chiryo, rub the spinal column from below to above).*

> Photos: 1 Forehead, 2 Temples, 3 Back of head, 6 On the head, 23 Heart, 24 Liver, 68 Pancreas, 7 Stomach and intestines, 55 Kidney area, 28 Bladder area, 57 Healing technique Hanshin Chiryo 1, 58 Healing technique Hanshin Chiryo 2, 59 Healing technique Hanshin Chiryo 3, 60 Healing technique Hanshin Chiryo 4, 61 Healing technique Hanshin Chiryo 5

Obesity: The heart, the kidneys, the stomach and intestines, the half of the body *(Hanshin Chiryo).*

> Photos: 23 Heart, 55 Kidney area, 7 Stomach and intestines, 57 Healing technique Hanshin Chiryo 1, 58 Healing technique Hanshin Chiryo 2, 59 Healing technique Hanshin Chiryo 3, 60 Healing technique Hanshin Chiryo 4, 61 Healing technique Hanshin Chiryo 5

Gout: The heart, the kidneys, the bladder, the stomach and intestines, the *Tanden*, the affected body area(s).

> Photos: 23 Heart, 55 Kidney area, 28 Bladder area, 7 Stomach and intestines, 31 Tanden

Heatstroke: The head area, the heart, the chest area, the stomach and intestines, the kidneys, the *Tanden.*

> Photos: 1 Forehead, 2 Temples, 3 Back of head, 6 On the head, 23 Heart, 22 Lungs—also cover the chest area, 7 Stomach and intestines, 55 Kidney area, 31 Tanden

– 7 –
Functional Disorders of the Urogenital Tract

(In the following chapter, the kidneys are included as a hand position under every health disorder. I leave my hands in this one position for at least ten minutes. Both hands on the kidneys warm the entire body.)

Nephritis (Kidney Inflammation):

The kidneys, the heart, the bladder, the stomach and intestines.
    Photos: 55 Kidney area, 23 Heart, 28 Bladder area, 7 Stomach and intestines

Pyelitis (Inflammation of the Pelvis of a Kidney):

The kidneys, the bladder, the *Tanden*.
    Photos: 55 Kidney area, 28 Bladder area, 31 Tanden

Renal Calculus (Kidney Stones):

The kidneys, the stomach and intestines, the bladder, the painful body area(s).
    Photos: 55 Kidney area, 7 Stomach and intestines, 28 Bladder area

Urosepsis:

The head area, the eyes, the stomach and intestines, the heart, the kidneys, the bladder, the *Tanden*.
    Photos: 1 Forehead, 2 Temples, 3 Back of head, 6 On the head, 8 Eyes, 7 Stomach and intestines, 23 Heart, 55 Kidney area, 28 Bladder area, 31 Tanden

Cystitis (Inflammation of the Bladder):

The kidneys, the bladder.
    (Drink at least two quarts of water every day. Keep your bladder warm with a pillow, blanket, or hot-water bottle. Treat the bladder directly for at least fifteen minutes; in acute, painful cases, until the pain has disappeared. Afterward, keep the bladder warm for at least one hour.)
    Photos: 55 Kidney area, 28 Bladder area

Urinary Calculus
(Bladder Stones):   The kidneys, the bladder, the painful area(s)of the body.
                Photos:55 Kidney area, 28 Bladder area

Bedwetting: The head area, on the head, the bladder, the kidneys.
                Photos: 1 Forehead, 2 Temples, 3 Back of head, 6 On the head, 28 Bladder area, 55 Kidney area

When Urine Can't Flow
Because of Swollen
Prostate Gland):   The kidneys, the bladder, the ureter
                Photos: 55 Kidney area, 28 Bladder area, 40 Ureter

---

– 8 –
Operation Wounds and Functional Disorder of the Skin

Wounds: The injured body area(s)—treat the body part without touching it until the pain is gone.

         (As already mentioned above, Dr. Usui recommends treating the affected body area until the pain has disappeared for all types of pain. For headaches, for example, treat the head; for backaches, treat the back. However, it is possible that a patient complains about back pain and the practitioner's hands automatically wander to another part of the body after the above-described Reiji. In this case, trust your hands more than the information your patient gives you! For all injuries, we mainly use the power symbol. As already mentioned, you can draw it on a piece of material, the bandage, or plaster cast—as long as it is not seen by a non-initiate.)

Contortions, Bruises,
Contusions: The affected body areas.

Inflammation of
the Lymph Nodes: The affected body areas, the *Tanden*.
                Photos: 31 Tanden

Broken Bones:

The affected body area(s)—(hands) above the plaster cast or bandage.

Splinters:

The affected body area(s).

Dislocated and Luxated Joints:

The affected body area(s).

Periostitis,
Ostitis (Inflammatory Bone Process),
Arthritis, Myositis
(Muscle Inflammation):

The affected body area(s), the *Tanden*.
    Photo: 31 Tanden

Muscular
Rheumatism:

The head area, the painful body area(s), the stomach and intestines—in order to regulate the bowel movement.
    Photos: 1 Forehead, 2 Temples, 3 Back of head, 6 On the head, 7 Stomach and intestines

Tuberculosis of the
Spinal Column:

The head area, the *Tanden*, the painful body area(s), the affected body area(s).
    Photos: 1 Forehead, 2 Temples, 3 Back of head, 6 On the head, 31 Tanden

Scoliosis:

The affected body area(s).

Syphilis of the
Spinal Column:

The head area, the *Tanden*, the painful body area(s), the affected body area(s).
    Photos: 1 Forehead, 2 Temples, 3 Back of head, 6 On the head, 31 Tanden

Dizziness, Fainting:

The heart, the head area—if the person has been rescued from drowning, only treat after the water has been expelled from the body.
    Photos: 23 Heart, 1 Forehead, 2 Temples, 3 Back of head, 6 On the head

Skin Rashes, Swelling,
(Skin)Tumors: The *Tanden*, the affected body area(s).
Photo: 31 Tanden

Nettle Rash: The stomach and intestines, the *Tanden*, affected body area(s).
Photos: 7 Stomach and intestines, 31 Tanden

Hair Loss: The head area, the stomach and intestines, the affected body area(s), the *Tanden*.
Photos: 1 Forehead, 2 Temples, 3 Back of head, 6 On the head, 7 Stomach and intestines, 31 Tanden

Leprosy: The head area, the stomach and intestines, the *Tanden*, affected body area(s), the half of the body *(Hanshin Chiryo)*.
(Should only be treated by a licensed physician.)
Photos: 1 Forehead, 2 Temples, 3 Back of head, 6 On the head, 7 Stomach and intestines, 31 Tanden, 57 Healing technique Hanshin Chiryo 1, 58 Healing technique Hanshin Chiryo 2, 59 Healing technique Hanshin Chiryo 3, 60 Healing technique Hanshin Chiryo 4, 61 Healing technique Hanshin Chiryo 5

Syphilis: The head area, the stomach and intestines, the *Tanden*, affected body area(s).
(Should only be treated by a licensed physician.)
Photos: 1 Forehead, 2 Temples, 3 Back of head, 6 On the head, 7 Stomach and intestines, 31 Tanden

– 9 –

Childhood Diseases

(Caution: Childhood diseases can become very critical for adults who did not have them as children!)

Nightly Weeping: The head area, the stomach and intestines.
(We suggest that children up to two-and-a-half years of age be taken into the parent's bed or have their bed placed directly next to the parent's. Small children aren't yet capable of dealing with nightmares

and states of fear. They need to be physically close to their parents, especially the mother at the beginning of life.)

> Photos: 1 Forehead, 2 Temples, 3 Back of head, 6 On the head, 7 Stomach and intestines

Measles:

The head area, the stomach and intestines, the heart, the affected body area(s).

> Photos: 1 Forehead, 2 Temples, 3 Back of head, 6 On the head, 7 Stomach and intestines, 23 Heart

German Measles:

As above.

> Photos: 1 Forehead, 2 Temples, 3 Back of head, 6 On the head, 7 Stomach and intestines, 23 Heart

Pertussis (Whooping-Cough):

The head area, the stomach and intestines, the heart, the lungs, the throat, beneath the sternum.

> Photos: 1 Forehead, 2 Temples, 3 Back of head, 6 On the head, 7 Stomach and intestines, 23 Heart, 22 Lungs, 5 Throat, 37 Beneath the sternum

Polio:

The head area, the stomach and intestines, the spinal column, the paralyzed affected body area(s).

> Photos: 1 Forehead, 2 Temples, 3 Back of head, 6 On the head, 7 Stomach and intestines, 57 Healing technique Hanshin Chiryo 1 (For this position and the next four, I recommend letting the hands rest in the individual positions until they move on their own to the next position. In case of doubt, stay in each position for five minutes.), 58 Healing technique Hanshin Chiryo 2, 59 Healing technique Hanshin Chiryo 3, 60 Healing technique Hanshin Chiryo 4, 61 Healing technique Hanshin Chiryo 5

Tonsillitis:

The affected body area(s).

– 10 –
Women's Health

Diseases of the Uterus:

The area of the uterus.
> Photos: 29 Area of the uterus, 30 Uterus, both sides, and ovaries

During Pregnancy:

Uterus: If the uterus is given treatment, the child will develop well and the birth will take place without complications.
> Photos: 29 Area of the uterus, 30 Uterus, both sides, and ovaries

The Birth:

The sacrum, the abdomen.
> Photos: 54 Sacrum, coccyx, 32 Genital organs

During Intense Morning Sickness:

The head area, the uterus, the stomach and intestines, beneath the sternum.
> Photos: 1 Forehead, 2 Temples, 3 Back of head, 6 On the head, 29 Area of the uterus, 30 Uterus, both sides, and ovaries, 7 Stomach and intestines, 37 Beneath the sternum

Diseases of the Breasts:

The breasts.

(I don't touch the breasts during treatment but keep my hands an inch or two above them. In my experience, there is a man in almost every seminar who exploits his Reiki abilities in this way.

If it is possible in terms of the culture, you can ask the affected patient beforehand whether she is comfortable with having your hands laid on her breasts. It is often easier for a woman to be touched by another woman.

As soon as a young girl's breasts begin to grow and constantly attract male attention, the breast area becomes armored as a form of protection. To counteract this process, my wife has developed a method of working with pressure in a shiatsu-like manner directly above and below the collarbone. This is also good for men!)
> Photo: 41 Breasts

64

Pregnancy Outside of the Uterus (Tubal Pregnancy):

The head area, the uterus, the painful body area(s).
> Photos: 1 Forehead, 2 Temples, 3 Back of head, 6 On the head, 29 Area of the uterus, 30 Uterus, both sides, and ovaries

– 11 –
Contagious Diseases

(Many of the following diseases are extremely contagious during a certain period of incubation. In no case should they be treated by laypeople during this time. Don't fool around with these diseases! Particularly in developing countries and crisis regions, some diseases that had almost died out during recent decades are now aggressively on the rise because antibiotics have been overused. Extreme caution is advised here. In any case, treatment should only be given by a licensed physician.)

Typhoid Fever:

The head area, the heart, the stomach and intestines, the pancreas, the *Tanden*—treat cautiously when there are complications.
When the disease has weakened the patient, it is possible that secondary health disorders will occur.
> Photos: 1 Forehead, 2 Temples, 3 Back of head, 6 On the head, 23 Heart, 7 Stomach and intestines, 68 Pancreas, 31 Tanden

Paratyphoid Fever:

As above.
> Photos: 1 Forehead, 2 Temples, 3 Back of head, 6 On the head, 23 Heart, 7 Stomach and intestines, 68 Pancreas, 31 Tanden

Dysentery:

The head area, the heart, the stomach and intestines, the *Tanden*
> Photos: 1 Forehead, 2 Temples, 3 Back of head, 6 On the head, 23 Heart, 7 Stomach and intestines, 31 Tanden

Dysentery in Children:

As above.
> Photos: 1 Forehead, 2 Temples, 3 Back of head, 6 On the head, 23 Heart, 7 Stomach and intestines, 31 Tanden

Diphtheria: The head area, the throat, the heart, the stomach and intestines, the kidneys, the *Tanden*. Anti-diphtheria serum is absolutely necessary (for successful treatment).

   Photos: 1 Forehead, 2 Temples, 3 Back of head, 6 On the head, 5 Throat, 23 Heart, 7 Stomach and intestines, 55 Kidney area, 31 Tanden

Cholera: The head area, the stomach and intestines, the heart, the *Tanden*.

   Photos: 1 Forehead, 2 Temples, 3 Back of head, 6 On the head, 7 Stomach and intestines, 23 Heart, 31 Tanden

Scarlet Fever: The head area, the mouth, the throat, the heart, the stomach and intestines, the kidneys, the *Tanden*, the affected (reddened) body area(s).

   Photos: 1 Forehead, 2 Temples, 3 Back of head, 6 On the head, 16 Over the mouth (don't close off lips), 5 Throat, 23 Heart, 7 Stomach and intestines, 55 Kidney area, 31 Tanden

**Flu
(Influenza Virus):**   The head area, the heart, the lungs, the stomach and intestines, the *Tanden*, the half of the body (Hanshin Chiryo), the painful body area(s).

   (For my part, I go to bed when I have the flu and practice being patient! High doses of up to 4 grams of Vitamin C per day and Echinacea drops are highly recommended.)

   Photos: 1 Forehead, 2 Temples, 3 Back of head, 6 On the head, 23 Heart, 22 Lungs, 7 Stomach and intestines, 31 Tanden, 57 Healing technique Hanshin Chiryo 1, 58 Healing technique Hanshin Chiryo 2, 59 Healing technique Hanshin Chiryo 3, 60 Healing technique Hanshin Chiryo 4, 61 Healing technique Hanshin Chiryo 5

**Epidemic, Cerebrospinal
Meningitis:**   The head area, back of neck, eyes, the heart, the stomach and intestines, the kidneys, the bladder, the spine—mainly the cervical vertebrae, the *Tanden*, the stiff or paralyzed area(s) of the body.

   Photos: 1 Forehead, 2 Temples, 3 Back of head, 6 On the head, 4 Back of neck, 5 Throat, 8 Eyes, 23 Heart, 7 Stomach and intestines, 55 Kidney area, 28 Bladder area, 57 Healing technique Hanshin Chiryo 1 (For this position and the next four, I recommend letting the hands rest in the individual positions until they move on their own to the next position. In case of doubt, stay in each position for five minutes and stay at the cervical vertebrae for ten minutes), 58 Healing technique Hanshin Chiryo 2, 59 Healing technique Hanshin Chiryo 3, 60 Healing technique Hanshin Chiryo 4, 61 Healing technique Hanshin Chiryo 5, 31 Tanden

Malaria:

The head area, the heart, the stomach and intestines, the liver, the pancreas, the *Tanden*. This treatment should be done one hour before the attack of fever.

> Photos: 1 Forehead, 2 Temples, 3 Back of head, 6 On the head, 23 Heart, 7 Stomach and intestines, 24 Liver, 68 Pancreas, 31 Tanden

Erysipelas:

The head area, the heart, the stomach and intestines, the *Tanden*, the affected body area(s)77.

> Photos: 1 Forehead, 2 Temples, 3 Back of head, 6 On the head, 23 Heart, 7 Stomach and intestines, 31 Tanden

Tetanus (Lockjaw):

The head area, the heart, the stomach and intestines, the *Tanden*, the injured body area(s), the painful body area(s).

> Photos: 1 Forehead, 2 Temples, 3 Back of head, 6 On the head, 23 Heart, 7 Stomach and intestines, 31 Tanden

Afterword

More than seventy years after Dr. Usui's death, the Reiki puzzle is in the process of completing itself before our astonished eyes. It is a great joy for me to be permitted to share this valuable information with all of you. I can't say why this honor was given to me. I was probably just simply at the right time and place with the right woman. More and more information by and about Dr. Usui is coming to light every day, and this is where the truth belongs. After all, Reiki stands for light and love. Many Reiki friends throughout the world continue to work toward spreading this light and this love all over the planet.

We are certain that the final word on the topic of Reiki and the history of Reiki has yet to be spoken. I definitely do not claim to be the ultimate authority. I am solely a tool in the hand of the Existence. In this sense, I bow in deep gratitude to Dr. Usui and to you.

I hope that you have enjoyed reading this book and that you use the techniques taught by Dr. Usui in your practice. This is the greatest joy for Dr. Usui and Reiki because you, my Dear Reader, are the hands of Dr. Usui.

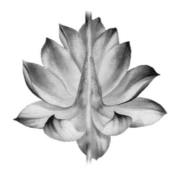

Original Japanese Texts

In response to requests by many people, some of the original Japanese texts are printed on the following pages. Since many of you cannot visit the impressive Usui memorial stone and let its beautifully radiant inscription have an impression on you, we have written it down for you here.

Don't worry—neither the publication of this text nor the photograph of the tombstone and memorial stone in any way violates any actual, moral-ethical, or unwritten Japanese law.

This memorial stone is located in a public cemetery in Tokyo and was set up there by the *Usui Reiki Ryoho Gakkai* so that it will be read. People don't erect memorials in the USA either when they want to keep a secret of something!

Even if most of you cannot decipher the characters (a skill that, unfortunately, has been kept from me as well), it is still a wonderful feeling to finally hold something by and about Dr. Usui in our hands.

Up to now, we in the West thought that Reiki was a so-called "oral tradition." It naturally lies in the nature of things that Reiki was mainly passed on through energy and words from the teacher to the student. But this doesn't exclude written language as a most important aid. Where would we be without the *Tao Te King*, *The Bible*, *The Upanishades*, the Buddhist *Sutras*, and *The Koran?* From world history, we know that oral traditions have often departed from this world together with their founders or at the latest after a few generations have passed. Fortunately, Dr. Usui was an extremely educated individual with a clear vision of the future. Moreover, he had perceived the nature of the human psyche and therefore took certain precautionary measures. In this way, his words have been preserved for us up to this present day.

Now here is the inscription of the memorial stone:

臼井先生功徳碑

修養錬磨ノ量ヲ積ミテ中ニ得ル所アルヲ之ヲ徳ト謂ヒ開導揆済シ人ニ施スヲ功ト謂フ功高ク徳大ニシテ始メテ一大宗師タルコトヲ得ヘシ古来ノ賢哲俊傑ノ士力學統ヲ空シ宗旨ヲ創メシ者ハ皆然ラサルナシ臼井先生ノ如キモ亦其ノ人ナルカ先生新ニ宇宙ノ靈氣ヲ本ツキテ心身ヲ善クスル法ヲ創メ四方伸々ニ開キ救ヒ乞ヒ摩ヲ顧ヒキ看創然トシテ之ヲ稱寛男二號ハ晩帆岐阜縣山縣郡谷合村ノ人其ノ先ハ八千年常胤ニ出ツ父俔字ハ衛門母ハ河合氏通稱字俔ヨリ苦學力行情篤キ超ユ長スルニ及ヒ歐米ニ航シ支那ニ游ケ電氣療法ヲ得タリ是ヨリ之ヲ身ニ試ミ人ニ驗スルニ功效立チトコロニ見ハレ先生慶應元年八月十五日ヲ以テ生レ昭和二年四月居ヲ東京青山原宿ニ定メ學會ヲ設ケ靈氣ヲ以テ鍛錬益々カスト大正十一年四月居ヲ東京青山原宿ニ定メ學會ヲ設ケ靈氣療法ヲ行フニ遠近来リ乞フ者戸外ニ溢ツ十一年九月大震火災起リ創傷病者到ル電ニ呻吟スルコト幾何ナルヲ知ルヘカラス其ノ急ニ患ヲ済フコト大平比ノ如シ後恵澤ヲ被ケ治療ヲ行フ逺近来リ之ヲ痛ミ日ニ出テ市ノ中外ニ業ス聲響鴉ハレ地方ヨリ招聘スル者少カラス急ニ應シ呉ニ之ヲ救ヘシ以テ十四年二月市ノ中外ニ業ス聲響鴉著ハレ地方ヨリ招聘スル者少カラス急ニ應シ呉ニ福山ニ入リ尋テ福山ニ抵ル偶疾作リ泰ニ客舎ニ殘ス時ニ大正十五年三月九日亨年六十二配鈴木氏名ハ貞子一男一女ヲ生ム男ハ不二ト曰ク家ヲ嗣ク女ハ慶ニ矯ル若キニ靈法ニ志スル所ハ止マラス宏島ニ入リ尋テ福山ニ抵ル偶疾作リ泰ニ客舎ニ殘ス時ニ大正十五年三月九日亨年六十二配鈴木氏名ハ貞子一男一女ヲ生ム二試ミ泉ニ功效立スルニ及ヒ歐米ニ航シ支那ニ游ケ電氣療法ヲ得タリ是ヨリ之ヲ身ニ試ミ人ニ驗スルニ功效立チトコロニ見ハレ先生出ツ父俔字ハ衛門母ハ河合氏通稱字俔ヨリ苦學力行情篤キ超ユ長スルニ及ヒ歐米ニ航シ支那ニ游ケ電氣療法ヲ得タリ是ヨリ之ヲ身ニ試ミ

故ニ其ノ人ヲ教フルヤ光ツ明天皇ノ遺訓ヲ奉體シ朝夕五戒ヲ唱ヘテ心ニ念シ今日恐ルレ勿レ憂フル勿レ業ヲ励メ人ニ親切ナレト是レ蓋シ修養ノ一大訓ニシテ逺慨古聖野ノ警戒スル者ト其ノ揆ヲ一ニセリ先生之ヲ以テ招福ノ祝法萬病ノ靈薬トナサハ其ノ本鋭ナル所知ラルヘシ而カモ其ノ修養法ハ極メテ卑近ヲ旨トシ何等高遠ノ事ナク靜生合掌瞑目朝夕念誦ノ際ニ醇健ノ心ヲ養ヒ平正ニ行フ復キ以テ爽健ニシテ運推移シ思想ヲ感動寄カラスこれを以て人生ノ福祉ヲ享ケシムルニ在リテ是レ靈法ノ世道人心ニ裨益スル所ナラン啻ニ病苦ヲ醫スルニ止マラス蓋シ本鋭ナル所知ラルヘシ而カモ其ノ修養法ハ極メテ卑近ヲ旨トシ何等高遠ノ事ナク靜生合掌瞑目朝夕念誦ノ際ニ醇健ノ心ヲ養ヒ平正ニ行フ者ニ比シ靈法ヲ普及セシムルハ其ノ世道人心ニ裨益スルナルハ何人モ企及シ易キニ非ス先生ノ靈能ニ因リテ心ヲ正シク身ヲ健ニシテ人生ノ福祉ヲ享ケシムルニ在リ靈法ノ世道人心ニ裨益スル所ナラン啻ニ病苦ヲ醫スルニ止マラス故ニ其ノ人ヲ教フルヤ光ツ明天皇ノ遺訓ヲ奉體シ朝夕五戒ヲ唱ヘテ心ニ念シ今日恐ルレ勿レ憂フル勿レ業ヲ励メ人ニ親切ナレト是レ蓋シ修養ノ一大訓ニシテ

二靈法ノ立トスル所ハ其ノ世道人心ニ裨益スルナルハ何人モ企及シ易キニ非ス先生ノ門ニ入ル者ニ比シ靈法ヲ普及セシムルハ其ノ世道人心ニ裨益スルナルハ何人モ企及シ易キニ非ス先生ノ靈能ニ因リテ心ヲ正シク身ヲ健ニシテ人生ノ福祉ヲ享ケシムルニ在リ是レ靈法ノ世道人心ニ裨益スル所ナラン先生ヤ資性温厚恭謙ニシテ邊幅ヲ飾ラス躯幹豊偉常ニ莞爾トシテ笑ヲ含ム事ニ當リヤ剛毅ニシテ克ク忍ヒ用意尤モ深シ善ク人ヲ勵メ五ヲ四二回々業ト勵メ五ヲ四二回々人ニ親切ナレト是レ蓋シ讀書ヲ好ミ史傳ニ渉リ修養ニ至ルマデ通セサルナシ且ツ醫薬経歴修養練磨ノ資料トナリ醫學經典ニ出入シ心理ノ學神仙ノ方術呪古聖相人ノ方術ニ至ルマデ一々力メテ卑近ヲ旨トシ何等高遠ノ事ナク靜生至ル所知ラルヘシ而カモ其ノ修養法ハ極メテ

二千餘人ヲ算フルニ至レリ此レ一ニ靈法ノ普及ヲ急務トセシニ因ル者ニ遠ク都下ニ道場ヲ會シテ逺東ヲ継キ地方ニ在ル者モ市名其ノ法ヲ傳フ先生斷クト雖トモ靈法ハ永久ニ世ニ宣播スヘシ者ニ遠ク都下ニ道場ヲ會シテ逺東ヲ継キ地方ニ在ル者モ市各其ノ法ヲ傳フ先生斷クト雖トモ靈法ハ永久ニ世ニ宣播スヘシ嗚呼先生ノ中ニ得テ外ニ施ス者ニ居キ門下ノ諸士相議シ石ヲ豊多摩郡西方寺ニ建チ其ノ功徳ヲ頌シ以テ不朽ヲ圖ラントシ文ヲ予ニ囑ス予深ク先生ノ偉頭ニ眼シ諸士ノ師率ノ誼ニ篤キヲ嘉ミシテ其ノ梗槩ヲ叙シ後人ヲシテ觀感瞻仰護ル能ハサラシメンコトヲ庶幾フ

昭和二年二月

従三位勲三等文學博士　岡田　正之　撰
海軍少将従四位勲三等功四級牛田従三郎書

中野町
石畑刻

◀ On the *left* is the inscription of the memorial stone that was erected next to Dr. Mikao Usui's grave.

▼ In the following, you will find a few pages of the original *Usui Reiki Ryoho Hikkei*, Dr. Usui's handbook. The pages 30 and 78 of this book also show the original pages describing the treatments. I hope this helps you get an idea of how it looked

This copy, which we received from T. Oishi, was printed instead of written in Dr. Usui's own handwriting. Unfortunately, we do not know whether there is a handwritten original.

公開伝授説明

肇祖 臼井甕男

古来能く独自の秘法を創見するや、己か子孫にのみ教えて家伝と為し之に依つて後世一門の生活安定を計り、秘法内容の門外不出を唱うるが如きは実に前世紀の遺習と申すもので、尚も現代の如く人類の共存共栄を以て幸福の基調となし、併せて社会の進歩を要望する時代に於ては、断じて一私するを許しません。我が臼井霊気療法は前人未発の創見でありまして、世上其比を見ません。されば之をば人間公益の為めに開放し、何人をも共に天恵に浴せしめ、以て霊肉一如を期し、人世天与の福祉を得しめんとするものであります。元より我が霊気療法は宇宙間の霊能に基く霊気の独創療法でありますから、此れに依つて先ず人間自體を壮健にし、思想の穏健と人世の愉悦を増進するのであります。

今や生活の内外に亘り、改善改造を要する秋に於て汎く同胞を悩める心と病災の裡より救うべく敢て公開伝授する所以であります。

Photo Appendix

All of the hand positions in Dr. Usui's *Original Reiki Handbook*

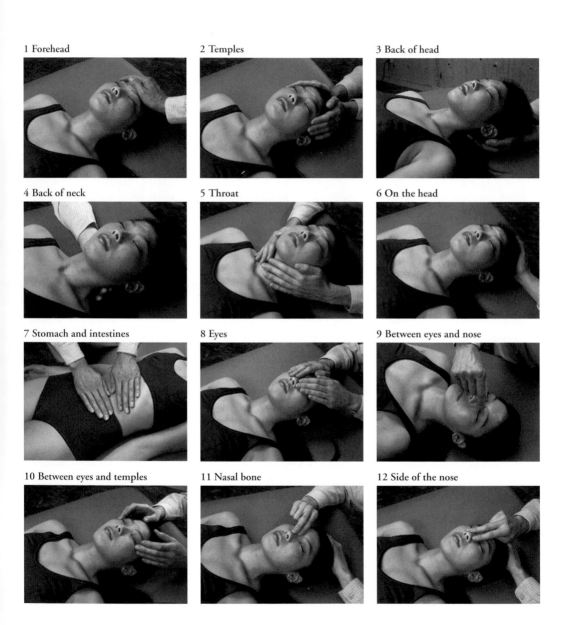

1 Forehead

2 Temples

3 Back of head

4 Back of neck

5 Throat

6 On the head

7 Stomach and intestines

8 Eyes

9 Between eyes and nose

10 Between eyes and temples

11 Nasal bone

12 Side of the nose

13 Middle of forehead

14 Auditory canal entering

15 In front of and behind ear

16 Over the mouth*

17 On the tongue**

18 Root of tongue**

19 Cartilage in throat

20 Middle of forehead

21 Middle of upper lips

22 Lungs

23 Heart

24 Liver

25 Large intestine—upper and side

26 Large intestine—below

27 Area of small intestine

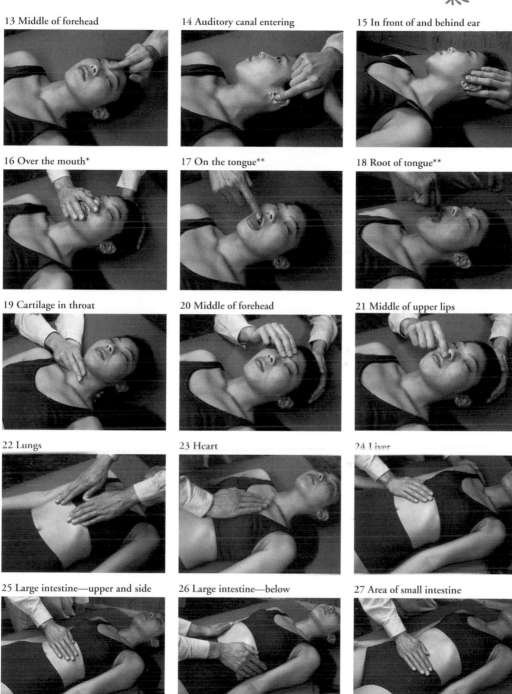

* Don't cover lips   ** Wear Latex gloves

28 Bladder area

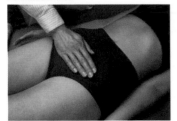

29 Uterus area

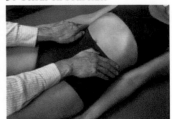

30 Uterus on both sides

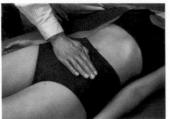

31 Tanden

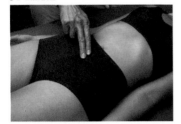

32 Genital organs

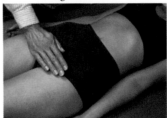

33 Diaphragm

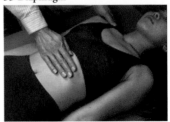

34 Windpipes

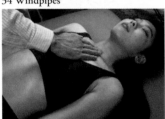

35 Bronchial tubes

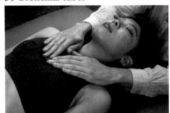

36 Heart area

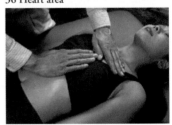

37 Below the sternum

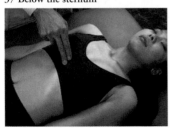

38 Appendix

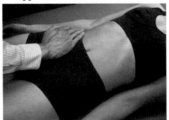

39 Abdominal area

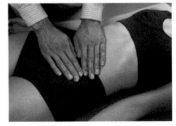

40 Ureter

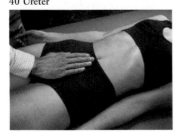

41 Breasts

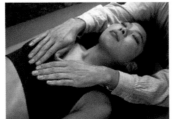

42 Cervical vertebra 1

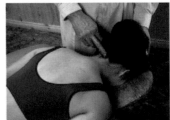

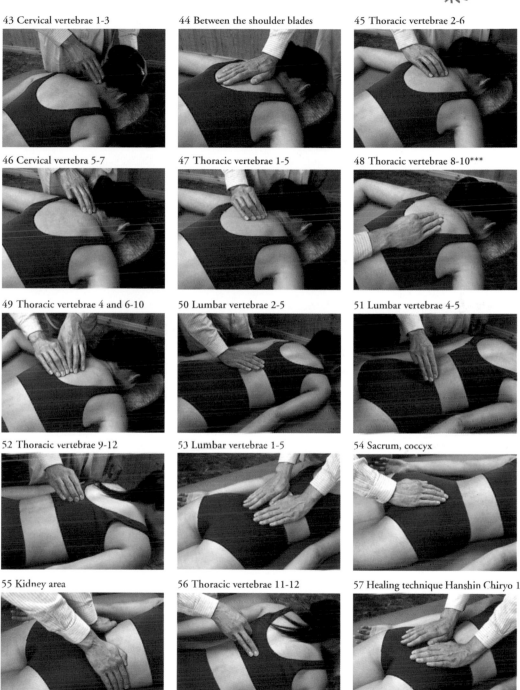

43 Cervical vertebrae 1-3

44 Between the shoulder blades

45 Thoracic vertebrae 2-6

46 Cervical vertebra 5-7

47 Thoracic vertebrae 1-5

48 Thoracic vertebrae 8-10***

49 Thoracic vertebrae 4 and 6-10

50 Lumbar vertebrae 2-5

51 Lumbar vertebrae 4-5

52 Thoracic vertebrae 9-12

53 Lumbar vertebrae 1-5

54 Sacrum, coccyx

55 Kidney area

56 Thoracic vertebrae 11-12

57 Healing technique Hanshin Chiryo 1

*** Mainly on right side

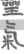

58 Healing technique Hanshin Chiryo 2

59 Healing technique Hanshin Chiryo 3

60 Healing technique Hanshin Chiryo 4

61 Healing technique Hanshin Chiryo 5

62 Cervical vertebrae 3-5

63 Elbows

64 Thumbs

65 Palms

66 Soles of feat

67 Anal area

68 Pancreas

69 Eyes heal

70 Breath heals

71 Massaging

72 Healing technique all****

****All fingertips of left hand

73 Tapping, fist

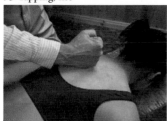

74 Tapping, fist

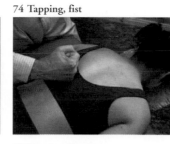

75 Tapping, fist

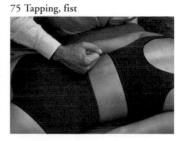

76 Tapping, fingers

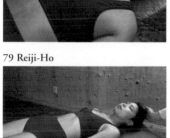

77 Tapping, fingers

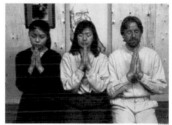

78 Tapping, fingers

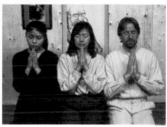

79 Reiji-Ho

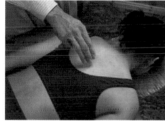

80 Gassho meditation

From left to right on photo 80:
Kumiko Kondo, Chetna Kobayashi, Frank Arjava Petter doing
the Gassho meditation.

Here is page 21 of the original book describing some of Dr. Mikao Usui's treatment positions.

靈氣療法必携

肝　胃　腸　　　膀　子

臟　　　　　　　胱　宮

二三四五胸椎

肝臟部、第八九十、胸椎（殊二右側）

胃部、第四六七八九十、胸椎

上行、横行、下行結腸部、小

腸部（臍附近）第六七八九十、

胸椎、第二三四五腰椎、臀部

膀胱部、第四五腰椎

子宮部及其両側、第九、十、十一、十二、

胸椎、第一二三四五腰椎、

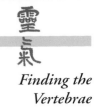

The spinal column is subdivided into seven cervical vertebrae, twelve
thoracic vertebrae, and five lumbar vertebrae. The first cervical vertebra
is located in the medulla oblongata, and the bottom one sticks out the
most at the lower end of the neck. You can easily find it by putting your
chin on your chest and feeling the back of your neck.

The first thoracic vertebra lies directly below it. The last thoracic
vertebra is at the point where the bottom rib meets the spinal column.
The lumbar vertebrae begin there and end at the sacrum. If you touch
your back while bending forward, you will notice where the bottom
lumbar vertebra is located.

The easiest way to find the cervical and thoracic vertebrae: find the
seventh cervical vertebra (Vertebra Prominens, also called C7) and go
from there two fingerwidths up or down along the spinal column. Not
everyone has a clearly defined spine of a vertebra.

The easiest way to find the lumbar vertebrae or the lower thoracic
vertebrae: Find the iliac crest (the uppermost bone of the pelvis above
the hip, at about the level of the navel). Follow a straight line from there
to the spinal column. Here you will find the fourth lumbar vertebra.
Move up or down the spinal column at a distance of 2.5 to 3
fingerwidths to find the other lumbar vertebrae or the lower
thoracic vertebrae. The distance to the lower thoracic vertebra is generally two fingerwidths.

The body of the vertebrae also has various sizes, according to an individual's body size.
Even a professional must count
the vertebrae.

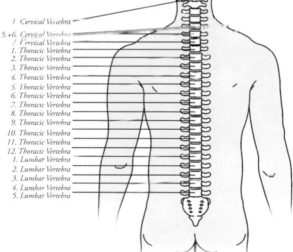

1 Cervical Vertebra
5.+6. Cervical Vertebra
7. Cervical Vertebra
1. Thoracic Vertebra
2. Thoracic Vertebra
3. Thoracic Vertebra
4. Thoracic Vertebra
5. Thoracic Vertebra
6. Thoracic Vertebra
7. Thoracic Vertebra
8. Thoracic Vertebra
9. Thoracic Vertebra
10. Thoracic Vertebra
11. Thoracic Vertebra
12. Thoracic Vertebra
1. Lumbar Vertebra
2. Lumbar Vertebra
3. Lumbar Vertebra
4. Lumbar Vertebra
5. Lumbar Vertebra

Reiki Music by Merlin's Magic

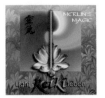
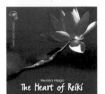

Merlin's Magic is a proven bestseller in the field of healing and relaxing music. The music of "Reiki", "Reiki - The Light Touch" and "The Heart of Reiki" was specifically composed and arrange to be played during Reiki treatments. Even for light relaxation, or for use therapuetically as background for massage or bodywork sessions of any kind, these recordings will delight you!

Reiki – The Light Touch
Sixty minutes of beautiful, serenely blissful instrumental music
CD $17.95* / ISBN 978-0-9102-6185-2
CASS $10.95*/ ISBN 978-0-9102-6179-1
INNER WORLDS MUSIC (60 min.)

The Heart of Reiki
Perfect accompaniment for Reiki treatment or body work sessions of any kind
CD $17.95* / ISBN 978-0-9102-6152-4
CASS $10.95* / ISBN 978-0-9102-6153-1
INNER WORLDS MUSIC (60 min.)

Healing Harmony
Harmonious, celestial compositions, best suited for supporting any type of healing
CD $17.95* / ISBN 978-0-9102-6150-2
CASS $ 10.95*/ ISBN 978-0-9102-6148-7
INNER WORLDS MUSIC (74 min.)

If you like to contact Frank Arjava Petter, please mail to:
arjava@reikidharma.com · www.reikidharma.com

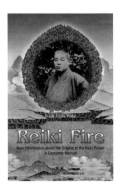
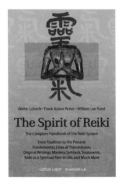
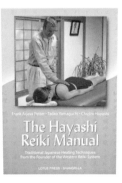
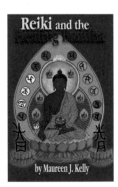

Frank Arjava Petter
Reiki Fire
New Information about the Origins of the Reiki Power
A Complete Manual
144 pages, $12.95
ISBN 978-0-9149-5550-4

Walter Lübeck, Frank Arjava Petter, William Lee Rand
The Spirit of Reiki
This is a handbook that reports on all the major aspects of Reiki in a concentrated and extensive manner.
312 pages, $19.95
ISBN 978-0-9149-5567-2

Frank Arjava Petter,
Tadao Yamaguchi,
Chujiro Hayashi
The Hayashi Reiki Manual
Dr. Hayashi Develped His Own Style Of Reiki And Became The Teacher Of Hawayo Takata, Who Introduced Reiki To The West.
112 pages, $19.95
ISBN 978-0-9149-5567-2

Mareen Kelly
Reiki and the Healing Buddha
Reiki and the Healing Buddha reconnects Reiki with its Buddhist – with new insights and viewpoints on Reiki.
216 pages, $15.95
ISBN 978-0-9149-5592-4

*SUGGESTED RETAIL PRICE